AF251664

Super Power

Super Power

Daniel Peter

Clovercroft Publishing

Published by Clovercroft Publishing, Franklin, Tennessee
ClovercroftPublishingGroup.com

Printed in the United States of America

ISBN: 978-1-956370-51-5 (print)

Contents

The Secret That Is Not So Secret

Why was this book written?

It is rare to find other men who understand how to use and wield their sexual power, how to apply sexual transmutation (which we will define more as this book goes on), or what we might call redirection. Most men I have known are depleted of sexual energy, enslaved by porn, and cannot control their sexual desires. And the men I knew who conquered their impulse to engage in sexual activity always associated sexual urges as something negative, or extremely negative.

After my own experience, and interviewing other men on their sexual recovery journeys, I have discovered new ways to wield sexual power in life and relationships. I am astounded by the massive benefits that can be gained in overcoming and using sexual power to enhance life.

I want to reach all men, especially those who don't know what to do and are about to give up on any attempt at sexual control. These men are ashamed to ask for help. I want to help people recover and encourage them to stop hiding their impulse.

My Story
(Part One)

After high school, I started asking questions. Why do religious practices teach people to abstain from sex before marriage, and why does sex have to be seen as only procreative? After wrestling with these thoughts for some time, I entered into a few romantic relationships while practicing abstinence. I noticed a big difference in these relationships versus sexual relationships, and I sought to find out why. I asked friends who practice abstinence in romantic relationships, and they saw the same differences. There was something there, and it was obviously different.

Next, I began to work on my addiction to pornography and masturbation. I read, studied, and attended sexual addiction (SA) meetings. This journey transformed me and others in such an empowering way that I had to share it. I was inspired by a good friend to start reading and dove deep into books about sex, masculinity, femininity, and sexual transmutation. This was when all my questions, and more, started to be answered. My eyes finally opened to the misconception of sex itself, and I started to gain answers on overcoming sexual addictions.

I would tell my friends I just had to write a book on this. I found only brief explanations of sexual power in books, and I knew I had to explain it more in-depth. The world is genuinely unaware of the power that sexual energy gives.

Glossary, or Definitions of Terms

What follows are some key terms I will use throughout this work. Note: this book will be frank. The terms are straightforward and unvarnished. I have ordered these not alphabetically, but in order of what I think will be most helpful with this book.

Sexual power: The force and potential behind sexual drive and energy.

Sexual energy: The energy behind sexual drive.

Sexual control: The ability to manage and control one's desire and attraction toward sex.

Sexual transmutation: The channeling of sexual energy into non-sexual activity, typically productive activity.

Sexual slavery: Enslavement to your own sexual desires.

Masculine power: The natural force of the male sex to influence tendencies like competition, aggression, and ambition.

Impulse: A sudden, strong, and unreflective urge or desire to act sexually.

The release: The escape of tension, specifically sexual tension, through ejaculation.

Depletion: The emptying oneself of sexual power through ejaculation.

Post-nut clarity: The clarity that is experienced after ejaculation.

Purpose: A man's objective in life, which gives him meaning and fulfillment.

Internal strength: Inner fortitude. The ability to withstand life's obstacles and continue to accomplish one's goals. This is within yourself; internal strength doesn't depend on anyone else.

Shit test: A manufactured grievance a woman uses to test the mettle, competence, and confidence of her mate.

High value man: This man is the epitome of masculinity, leadership, charm, and sophistication. He is a man of means and influence, loved by women, revered by men, and moves gallantly through the challenges of life with courage and pride.

Frame: This represents the plans, boundaries, and beliefs that a person carries. You can either step into someone else's frame or stay in your own.

Feminine: Is dynamic, passive, unpredictable, intuitive, caring, and heart-oriented. The polar opposite of the masculine, typically more naturally expressed in women.

Masculine: Is action-oriented, stable, predictable, logical, and focused. The polar opposite of the feminine, typically more naturally expressed in men.

Sub-personality: Natural identity patterns that emerge throughout a person's life that develop consciously or subconsciously.

Your edge: The threshold of growth and self-expansion.

My Story
(Part Two)

Where does my drive to write this book come from? It's rooted in my story.

I grew up in a Roman Catholic family where we lived under the presumption of abstinence. And yet we never talked about sex, pornography, or why abstinence was important.

I developed a pornography addiction in elementary school, and it was destroying me from the inside. I was ashamed and defeated. No matter what I did, I always went back to pornography. I prayed and prayed, but nothing happened.

I had literally thousands of hours sucked into the world of porn addiction, and I wouldn't dare tell my parents. In my teenage years I would ask others for help: friends, even Catholic priests. I took the advice they gave, which was to pray more and try harder, but nothing seemed to work. Others revealed that they also struggled with pornography. I was virtually hopeless in finding someone who had defeated their addiction.

I experienced sexual relationships, and these only made my addiction worse. I continued looking for help and began reading books and researching wherever I could. I became the guinea pig, and this was my experiment. I smashed electronic devices I used for pornography, I would put porn blockers on my computer, and I would journal and try to replace my addiction with those sorts of behaviors. Sometimes they seemed to work and sometimes they didn't. I would ask and analyze why. I found Sexaholics Anonymous, and finally other men who had been able to go without their addiction for durations of time. I found hope!

However, the answers they gave were not so tangible. The answer they most often gave was to just keep coming to groups. Why did this work? I continued to do my research and interviewed others about their experiences. I found patterns, and they were eye-opening.

Shortly after a sexual relationship, one of my partners got the disease of chlamydia. I didn't know if I had it; however, I took medication just in case. I was still on my father's health insurance at the time. I just hoped that he would never find out about the medication because my parents would then know I was having sex. One day while visiting my parents, my dad walks in surprised while looking at the mail. What an embarrassing—but necessary—moment.

My parents and I got real and would talk for hours about the matters of sex and abstinence. They never gave me an answer that made sense; however, I was inspired to look deeper into the matter. I found Pure in Heart in Boston and *Theology of the Body* by Saint John Paul II. The puzzle pieces were starting to come together, and my understanding of abstinence became obvious even for someone who is not a person of faith.

Once I was able to get control of my addiction, I began a relationship based on abstaining. The difference was profound. Instead of what I thought, and so many other men I know thought, the relationship didn't need sex, and we actually increased the attraction we had for each other. The relationship had something to it that made it more exciting. There was anticipation and excitement as well as a strong respect and honor for each other. I kept looking further into the matter, discovering, more and more, the logic and reasoning behind abstinence.

During this period I was introduced to the "red pill community." This refers to the truth about reality, especially a truth that is difficult to accept. This community would not support pornography; however, ironically, it supported promiscuous sex.

The relationship benefits I had with myself and others were much better. I read *Think and Grow Rich* by Napoleon Hill and his chapter on sexual transmutation. Who knew there can be so much power beyond the human desire for sex? I enjoyed it, but like many of the books I have read on sex and addiction, it wasn't tangible and was missing too many details.

While recovering, I noticed a change in attitude about my life and goals. My energy level and ambition to achieve goals increased. I found that other men would notice significant, positive differences as well. I knew other men needed to know and understand this just as I have.

I quickly realized that nobody talks about this subject, and I found out how hard it was to find men free from their addictions. The fact that nobody talked about it around me left me helpless and uninformed when I was younger.

I didn't want other men to feel the same. I didn't want other men to never understand the true power behind their addiction. These are the true reasons I have written this book.

—*Daniel Peter*

One

Sexual Energy and Sexual Power

If you don't control your balls, your balls will control you.

We drastically underestimate the power of sex and sexual energy. When a male is sexually aroused, a massive amount of energy surges through his body until the climax, which results in ejaculation. The energy that once was there is now gone. Males have vast amounts of sexual energy pulsing through their bodies, ready to release at nearly any moment. Men didn't choose this sexual power; it chose them.

If you doubt the power of this sexual energy, it is because you haven't consciously witnessed it. Have you fully resisted your sexual urges, or have you even come close? You won't feel the flow of this energy until you

> YOU WON'T FEEL THE FLOW OF THIS ENERGY UNTIL YOU STAND AGAINST IT. YOU CANNOT MEASURE ITS FORCE UNTIL YOU OVERCOME IT.

stand against it. You cannot measure its force until you overcome it. You cannot accurately measure anything unless you apply greater resistance to it.

Energy is power, or at least potential power. This energy is at your disposal if you can get a hold on it. It has the power to take action to create and produce. Although it may come from one source, it expresses itself in many forms.

This is a book for men. This is not a book to disempower women, but instead is one to better understand men—sometimes by relating them to women. The first half of this book will be about understanding the male sexual drive and the benefits of abstinence; the second half will be about overcoming and redirecting the male sexual drive.

Even though men and women are equal beings, they are very different. One of the differences between men and women is their natural hormones. Before advanced technology, men and women were valued for their natural gifts. Both sexes brought unique talents and gifts to their families and community. They were looked to for their strengths. Their strengths gave them purpose, and purpose made them feel fulfillment and importance.

Just some of the natural gifts of women include nurturing, intuition, caring, connecting, empathy, and many more.

The natural gifts of men include being action-oriented, aggressive, assertive, competitive, ambitious, driven, and more.

In traditional roles in society, women took care of the home, the children, and the community.

Men protected the borders, hunted for food, and fought off enemies.

Yes, men can have some of a woman's attributes, and women can have some of a man's attributes. However, this does not come naturally. This isn't a battle about gender; this is an understanding of the facts of sexual urges and hormones in men. A man's tendencies are associated with masculinity, and a woman's tendencies are associated with femininity. These are essentially polar opposites. Opposites tend to attract and contribute to a relationship.

You may say that since we are in a time of physical peace and technological advancement, we don't need those attributes. The truth is that we need them more than ever. (I will explain this later in the book.)

A man's sexual urges are not the same as a woman's.

Let's stop for a note: in some selected places in this book, I will use the word *fuck*. There is a reason. The word *sex* does not emulate a man's sexual urge like the word fuck. This urge is impulsive and powerful. It is wild and ruthless in nature.

Women can have strong sexual urges; however, men's urges are different. Men will face an overpowering spontaneous sexual force to fuck. It doesn't just go away; it lingers. It is strong, you can feel its strength, and most men in many environments cannot control it and must release it.

Men can fuck without being tiresome. A man's sexual drive has so much stamina that, during a sexual encounter, the man almost always neither stops to catch his breath nor gets distracted by physical fatigue. The urge for sex can control a man to the point in which he will either do something he will regret or even have sex with someone or something, an act he will regret.

Sexual energy doesn't look for love and connection; sexual energy looks to fuck and to fuck only. Sexual energy doesn't think. It acts, it does, it accomplishes. Like the adrenal glands, which inspire you to fight or flight. No thinking, or inaction, is involved. It is like a bull out of control. It is like energy with a mind of its own. It is uncontrolled power.

Do not reject your sexual urges. Instead, embrace them, for they enhance the human body, mind, and spirit. Of course, we must release that energy, but how we release it makes all the difference.

Men: without your balls, you wouldn't be the same.

A man's testicles produce 95 percent of the body's testosterone. Physical (or chemical) castration has the following symptoms: weight gain, muscle loss, fatigue, and reduced aggression.

"Destroy the sex glands, whether in man or beast, and you have removed the major source for action; for proof of this, observe what happens to any animal after it has been castrated. A bull becomes as docile as a cow after it has been altered sexually. Sex alteration takes out of the male, whether man or beast, all the fight that was in him."
–NAPOLEON HILL, *THINK AND GROW RICH*

Male animals fight each other and become aggressive. This is all dependent on testosterone. Even a mostly peaceful animal like the red deer will periodically show aggressive behavior toward each other. Castrate the red deer and this behavior does not happen. Supplement the castrated dear with testosterone, and this behavior returns.

The testosterone that men produce plays a crucial role in creating this sexual energy.

"This is evidenced in our own hormonal biology; healthy men possess between 12 and 17 times the amount of testosterone (the primary hormone in sexual arousal) women do, and women produce substantially more estrogen (instrumental in sexual caution) and oxytocin (fostering feelings of security and nurturing) than men."
–ROLLO TOMASSI, *THE RATIONAL MALE*

Testosterone increases your energy. Emotion, action, and living are a release of energy. All energy is directed. Energy cannot be destroyed, only redirected. It has potential. This potential is power, and we have the choice of how to use that power.

Not every man has access to all of his potential sexual power. Instead, the power that most men possess has been drained by modern-day stimuli, sex, porn, masturbation, lack of self-control, and virtual reality.

Men have great power and yet, for the most part, only know how to get *rid* of that power. Nobody has taught these men the truth of their gifts and power. Nobody has taught them how to redirect this force into something more.

The nerd uses the same sexual energy that the warrior fighting in a battle uses, just in different ways. We were designed like the animals of the earth, but we have the ability and capabilities to do so much more.

What kind of power are we talking about? This power can turn a man into an insane beast. Sexual energy with other emotions involved can cause a great deal of damage. Napoleon Hill calls this mix of emotions and sex "chemistry of the mind." A man motivated by sex will go to great heights for a woman. The confidence, mission, and strength are all gone when a man "falls in love." Love can cripple a man, but is it really love? No, it's the desire for sex. Men don't just fall in love. Their goal is sex with the one, or ones, they desire. They want it so bad they will give up things that are important to them. The desire for sex is an incredible force. Men have a hard time loving from afar. You may have seen men so obsessed with a woman that, as a result, they change their behavior and will do anything to have her. You may have heard these men described as "weak" or their actions as "approval-seeking behavior." This is power, and the woman who is desired is sucking that power out of him. She is in control, and she can manipulate. His intense, desiring thoughts burn up all his sexual energy. His intense focus and fantasies are a big part of his time, energy, and power.

This is like an inefficient car burning way more fuel than it needs to run. That fuel is going somewhere, but it's not going to get you to your destination. Before you know it, you'll have an empty gas tank and cannot drive to your next location. It's a waste of gas, a waste of time, and a waste of money. So is the man who is sexually depleted. He has no power, little energy, and now is wasting time.

Sexual energy combined with jealousy can be an unimaginable mix. These can cause anger, rage, aggression, and motivation for revenge.

Most men don't just fly by the seat of their pants; they fly by the desire of their balls. This is where ambition comes from. When a man sees a woman and is attracted to her, it's not about talking to her and taking her out for some fun. It's about having sex with her. You can hide your desire, but the desire is there, and at certain times it is much stronger than other times.

When men have a strong desire for sex, they become highly motivated.

> *"Sex desire is the most powerful of human desires."*
> –NAPOLEON HILL, *THINK AND GROW RICH*

Have you ever gone without sex or masturbation for a month? How about two weeks? Can you feel a change? The desire for sex has increased, and your sexual energy has recharged. Many men have never experienced what it's like to have all that sexual energy from abstaining for that amount of time. When men hit their peak of containing this power/sexual energy and cannot control or redirect it, they have to release it—most of the time in an uncontrollable way. Men become aroused by things they weren't aroused by before. Men feel like they need to release that energy, that they cannot contain it. They do not have control. When this happens, men become aggressive, hyper-focused, energized, even creative. Once they ejaculate and release all their energy, they become calm like a beast that has been tamed.

Sometimes men will have sex with their female friends whom they are not particularly attracted to, and only after finishing and releasing their load do they regret what they were so focused on. And sometimes men will have sex with other men. This is not for love; this is for the release.

Sexual energy is all about the mission and the goal. It does not think about right and wrong. Post-nut clarity is when you ejaculate and instantly see your situation differently, usually regretting this past action. You no longer have a sexual urge due to the energy that you depleted, as well as the hormones rushing through your body. Once you ejaculate, new hormones are released, and these make you docile. The sexual energy in your brain that was consuming your thoughts and intentions to fuck and fuck only is now gone. You view what you did as though somebody else made you do it. That is the power of sexual energy.

I am not saying that women can't experience this power; however, it exists in men to a much higher degree.

Women fight with words; men fight with fists. Women and men do not operate the same way.

Women can fight with fists, and men can fight with words; however, it is more common and natural for men to fight physically, expressing their energy in that way. Men may have an underlying desire to fight and wrestle. This sexual energy creates that desire to compete, be dominant, and exert power. It will increase a man's will to win and stamina to keep fighting.

Men bond through doing, and women bond by talking. A man's sexual power makes it natural to do something and to physically move. Men don't build as much rapport communicating as women do. A man can play hours of video games with other men without much communication, and at the end they will feel they have built a relationship. There are other aspects to how this works. In the end, a man's sexual energy is action-oriented, so when a man sees someone demonstrating an action, he can relate. Men build rapport by showing similarities.

Look at a group that consists only of men. These groups look much different than groups of women. These groups have a purpose and mission. They develop ranks, leadership, and hierarchy. Codes and conduct. These groups of men are driven toward their goals and can become outrageous and violent. Look at gangs, militaries, fraternities. Most of these groups are filled with out-of-control sexual power. Sexual power enlightens the group to the point that it becomes natural to bond and achieve more, whether good or bad, than could have been accomplished alone. This is the power of sexual energy.

In *The Way Of Men*, Jack Donovon talks about forming a fraternity and says, "That said, don't start trying to figure out your colors or your secret handshake just yet. These kinds of male cultural phenomena will occur organically as the result of shared history and identity."

This can be a curse. However, it can also be a tool to make men powerful.

"The emotion for sex is an 'irresistible force' against which there can be no opposition as an 'immovable body.' When driven by this emotion, men become gifted with a superpower for action."
–NAPOLEON HILL, *THINK AND GROW RICH*

We were built for survival. Human psychology is made to protect and adapt. This is why children develop "wounds from the past." Children learn to act in certain ways to protect themselves, physically or mentally, from the past. The brain is powerful and has adapted to survive and fill whatever needs were necessary at the time. The new patterns created are like an unstoppable force unless they are worked through, and taken seriously in doing so. This is just one example of the power of human psychology.

OVERCOME THE URGE, AND YOU WILL LEARN TO OVERCOME MUCH MORE. JUST LIKE WHEN A FATHER TEACHES HIS SON HOW TO GET BACK UP WHEN HE IS KNOCKED DOWN, OVERCOMING YOUR URGE TEACHES YOU HOW TO OVERCOME OTHER OBSTACLES IN LIFE.

While comfort decreases our ability to function, discomfort increases our ability to perform. A muscle doesn't grow without tension, nor does a man grow without challenge.

Our sexual urges are not only for a man to redirect into power and energy but are the foundation of a man's growth in strength. Some men may struggle more than others; however, we all experience the urge. Overcome the urge, and you will learn to overcome much more. Just like when a father teaches his son how to get back up when he is knocked down, overcoming your urge teaches you how to overcome other obstacles in life. The ripple effect is compounding. The strength, self-awareness, and experience are there for you when you face challenges in the future. When men overcome their urges, they make more money, more friends, and ultimately have a more abundant life. So will you when you have overcome your urge.

In *Hard Times Create Strong Men,* Stefan Aarnio writes, "Nonetheless, sexual transmutation is important, and I have personally used sexual transmutation in my most successful times in my life. The first time I practiced it, I made $42,000 in a week and wrote a book in 30 days."

Animals will fuck when they have the urge to fuck and eat when they have the urge to eat. They do not have a choice. Suppose you put healthy, nourishing meat in front of a starving dog. The dog will devour it as fast as possible. Dogs, like other animals, react to instinct. That dog doesn't have a choice; men have a choice. You can either stoop to the level of animals by letting your sexual urges gain control over you, or you can become more by gaining control over your sexual energy. You have a choice. When men gain control over their sexual urges, they can redirect that energy and power toward recreating their destinies.

Two

Women in Relation to the Sexual Power of Men

*There isn't a war on men; there is a war on the power
that men possess. Power is neither good nor evil;
whoever wields that power determines its destiny.*

You, as a man, are already biologically powerful. Besides your ability to move and create, you have much to give because of the deep urges inside you. When referring to power, I am referring to the unique motivation, inspiration, and energy men have, often directly triggered by sex. Power is only potential; strength, however, is the measure of your ability to direct such power.

When women sense weak men, they test their strength. Testing is a subconscious reaction from women. It's like when your brother teases you, and you take it personally and get mad. Your brother would have had more respect for you if you didn't take it personally. Acting this way would demonstrate emotional strength. The world will always test men for their strength. Why? Because, as humans, we inherently seek security. When shit hits the fan, men are the ones who fight the wars and clean up the messes. Physical strength is important, but emotional strength always comes first. If you are unable to use your emotional strength to face fear or say no to a threat, physical strength is useless. Men have power but do not always control it. A weak man is not powerless. He just doesn't control his power.

> MEN HAVE POWER BUT DO NOT ALWAYS CONTROL IT. A WEAK MAN IS NOT POWERLESS. HE JUST DOESN'T CONTROL HIS POWER.

The strength role has to be filled. When women see that men are not taking this role, they try to take it themselves. When women sense weakness in men, they learn not to trust men. This trust isn't the same as trusting a friend with your bank account. This trust is about having self-accountability, leading and confidently making decisions in one's own life, and not giving your agency to anyone else. She can't trust you to hold your own and not depend on her. Women, and the feminine, subconsciously understand the need for this strength for security. The feminine needs the masculine just as much as the masculine needs the feminine. Polarity in homosexual relationships is an example of this. Even in a same-sex relationship one partner tends to be more masculine and the other more feminine. It is balance, and the roles must be filled in order for the relationship to function well.

When women cannot rely on men, they can only rely on other women and/or themselves. That is why you see women taking up masculine roles in the household. The feminist movement is a result of women attempting to fill the need for strength. A woman's goal in this case is either to fill a man's role and or to access power.

If you are perceived as weak, the woman in your life may feel she cannot trust you and what you have to offer. She sees that you are led by emotion and not by beliefs. She senses your weakness and unreliability because emotions can easily change. Even if your emotions are

IF YOU ARE PERCEIVED AS WEAK, THE WOMAN IN YOUR LIFE MAY FEEL SHE CANNOT TRUST YOU AND WHAT YOU HAVE TO OFFER. for her, she will not appreciate the genuineness of it. A strong man is genuine when his beliefs are aligned with his actions, not when his emotions are aligned with his actions.

Women naturally need some kind of strength, so they choose to become the strength you are supposed to be. They will deplete you of your power because your power can get in the way of her ability to fill her need for strength. A couple struggling to get by, even just to survive, must fill their roles in a relationship. Two butting heads is inefficient and ineffective. Someone needs to be the leader, and if she can't trust your strength, she will make herself the leader. An example of this is the men who change and become docile and indecisive after getting married and give this role to their wife.

Do not blame women for reacting the way they are reacting. Their reaction is a natural one, the result of not having safety and security. It is not in a woman's nature to be strong or be a leader. A woman may try to fill the gap when men do not fill that role, but she is unlikely to feel efficient and happy in this position. She does not have access to the natural masculine sexual energy that men do. Women cannot create that power, so they have to take it from men. If someone has something that you don't have, you are at a disadvantage. But when you take away that something that they have, there is no more disadvantage. Women don't create sexual masculine power; they take it away from men or manipulate men to use their power.

Before we go further, let me provide two definitions of power from the Merriam-Webster dictionary.

1. the ability to act or produce an effect

2. possession of control, authority, or influence over others

Women will use your power (the ability to act or produce an effect, that is influenced and enhanced by your sexual drive) if they don't trust you with it. They will test you with bait and use it to influence you. Most weak men today need and want women more than women want and need them. Men "need" and "want" women for sex and approval for sex. It gives men a sense of freedom and certainty that they can stabilize their sexual "need" and feed their self-esteem. Either way, a woman will have more power with a man because the man is emotionally strong, and she can lean on his power. If it's not being shown by the man, the woman can take his power by taking advantage of his energetic drive and turning it into action that can get her things she would have a hard time getting on her own, if at all, including non-physical things like attention and affirmation.

Relationship happiness and approval is indirectly aligned with access to sex. In a weak man's mind a bad relationship and disapproval is equal to no sex. Women test both strong and weak men, and the difference is the way the man responds. When a woman senses a weak man, all she has to do is toy with the idea of sex with him, or the standing of their relationship, and she knows he will bite. Whoever needs the other most will compromise the most.

THERE IS A POWER DYNAMIC IN RELATIONSHIPS WHETHER WE LIKE IT OR NOT.

There is a power dynamic in relationships whether we like it or not. The hierarchical nature among humans will always come into effect.

In 2022 I parked my car on a Boston street. It was 8 o'clock, and it was still light out because it was the middle of summer. I walked by a store on the street and looked through the window. There I saw an ugly doll sitting on a shelf; it had these words on its chest:

"When ya got 'em by the balls, their hearts and minds will follow."

This quote rings true both literally and figuratively. Something has you by the balls. What could it be?

A man's sexual power can be accessed through pleasure, fantasy, accomplishment, status, and most of all, sex.

Women play a huge role in this power because all high-sexed men want sex, and most men want sex with a feminine woman. The same power is not within a woman, however. Women, through their unique inner sense of being more intuitive, mostly subconsciously, sense this dynamic in men, and know what they desire.

Women have leverage on men, but that is only because men allow them to have it. Men are motivated both by the sex they can have as well as the sex they miss out on. This is a powerful combination.

Men will go to great heights for women. Men will go to great heights for sex. Men will take women out on fancy vacations, buy expensive jewelry, change laws, break their morals for women, and much more. Women don't have the same type of power, but they can redirect a man's biological power to achieve their own goals. Most men think sex is negotiable. It's only negotiable when dealing with a prostitute. Negotiable sex is possible, but never genuine. Women take full advantage of this. Men think the more they do for a woman, the more likely it is that she will have genuine sex with them—or any sex at all.

> MOST MEN THINK SEX IS NEGOTIABLE. IT'S ONLY NEGOTIABLE WHEN DEALING WITH A PROSTITUTE. NEGOTIABLE SEX IS POSSIBLE, BUT NEVER GENUINE.

This is false. The opposite will occur, and overdoing it for a woman actually makes it less likely that she will have sex with you. All it does is reveal emotional weakness. Misuse of power is not actual power; it is potential power that has been wasted. Women will take advantage of your power and then leave without giving the reward of sex. You will find out that women do not think like men. From a man's point of view, women are illogical. Understand the feminine point of view, and you will understand women. To women, men are only true men *in the moment.* Whatever good you did for a woman years ago or even a few days ago does not matter. It's about right now. Power in the past doesn't matter. Power matters *now.* All men have that power whether they use it or lose it. A man's willingness to go to great heights for a woman by doing unnecessary, over-the-top things for her shows her the value and strength of his power. This shows her that as soon as he gets it he will waste it. Power is not strength if it is not under control and under your command. The potential is there, but without a strong commander and leader, the potential has no purpose and is useless. This is just like an army with no captain which is, in reality, lacking any purpose. Therefore, the army is not a threat and has no actual power.

Approval-seeking behavior is an indirect motive for sex, and this leads to men letting their power be abused by women they seek sex from. Men will try to bribe a woman and bend over backwards for them to gain their favor. In giving in to the impulse, approval "ensures a better chance of sexual release." This will make men "feel" like they have the right to sex and that the woman is obligated to give it to him. The fantasy of earning this approval can drive men insane. Men will have anxiety about saying and doing the "perfect" things to earn a woman's favor. Men may not admit it, but their actions are driven by this approval.

It is not that women will want to access your power. They are not evil. They *want to be led* by strength and power, and if they are not led by a man in this way, they will take and manipulate to use that power in ways that benefit them. It may be hard at first because a woman wants to be sure of your strength will and keep testing you. Obviously, don't be tyrannical with your leadership—that only shows weakness as well. Tyrannical leadership, at first, can look like strength, but it only comes from underlying weakness and insecurity.

Women are attracted to power. *Hypergamy* is proof of this. One of the most common definitions for *hypergamy,* which I will use here, is the action of marrying or forming a sexual relationship with a person with a superior sociological or educational background. Women are attracted to men who have the most strength, status, riches, education—things of this sort. All this is power. It is a form of masculine and sexual power. Also, it is rooted in the biology of women to find a man of high status because it guarantees her survival as well as that of her offspring. Women are attracted to these kinds of men because they have the highest amount of potential sexual power and have proven it through acquiring success in life. It's like choosing the fastest car on the lot. The driver has the *potential* to drive the fastest only if he knows how to drive the car. It isn't quite that simple with accessing sexual power. However, it is a similar concept.

There are two ways women use the sexual power in a man. One is by manipulating men by using their desire for sex against them, which we've talked about in this chapter. The second? I will discuss it in the next chapter. It is through weakening a man of his sexual power by depletion.

The definition of "highly sexed" is: having strong sexual urges.

Not all men are highly sexed men, especially when they have low testosterone.

Three

The Misuse of Male Sexual Power in Culture

There are three ways that culture functions regarding high-sexed men. A culture has all three, but one of them usually outweighs the other two.

The first way of functioning in culture is through imagination: a high-sexed man's power is hijacked through fake sex and competition. The power is used in an unproductive way through virtual reality and entertainment.

The second way of functioning is through imitation: a man's power is expressed, unleashed, and out of control through promiscuous sex, violence, cults, gangs, and crime.

The third way of functioning is through a rational outlet: the man's power is redirected in a productive way. Ambitious men, those who are high achievers, running businesses, or are hardworking, and physically strong men.

The causes for these cultural functions can vary. War, hard times, and poverty can sometimes have a positive effect and influence men to be productive with this power. Abundance and peace can also often influence men to be unproductive and direct their power through imagination or irrational action. There are other factors as well, like the access to sex and entertainment. Tyrants and chaotic leadership can influence men to amplify and waste this power. And older men can influence younger men through the use and productive amplification of this power.

Sexual power *will* find a way to escape. The question is how. The nature of sexual power is to act and react. Only the wielder of that power can be proactive and redirect it into conscious action. Sexual power will find a way to release itself in the most pleasurable and effortless way. It does not comprehend; it just *does*. The closest and most readily available way to release it is usually with little thought. The owner of the power will feel a strong pull toward what will be the releasing agent.

A man's sexual power does not come with morals; its nature is to expand, grow, accomplish, and achieve. All the desires and tendencies ensure survival. Men were built to always be fighting to survive, and sex is at least one place where this fight comes from. Sexual power can be displayed and emulated in different ways that are not through sex. It has a procreative nature: sex is meant to create life that can drive men to physically create. It has a survivability nature: it draws out the desire to survive and compete for a partner. Last, sex's impulse-oriented nature brings out the desire to move and act.

Progress, accomplishment, and achievement use the procreative nature of this power. Challenge, competition, and personal status use the survivability nature of this power. Mission, goals, and purpose use the impulse for potential action that sexual power craves.

This is why it is hard for highly sexed males to sit still in classrooms, play with dolls, or indulge in romantic novels. This isn't just a craving, this is a vigorous, energetic impulse yearning to be released and put to work.

Gangs, cults, and even religions take sexual power and compound its use. These organizations put sexual power into one goal. Competitiveness can be a factor here, but procreative power is used for the purpose of creating or reproducing something.

Men use sexual power in hard times, poverty, and war in a way that moves them to face challenges. These events bring about the sexual power of survival. Sexual power's goal is to gain status and importance to ensure survival.

A man's use of sexual power doesn't know the difference between what is real and what is fake.

What would the feminist do without video games and pornography? Men have voluntarily castrated themselves. We tell kids to not be lured in by older men in a van with candy—and rightly so, in every way—but we don't teach boys to avoid the more subtle kidnappers of their lives. Sex is candy for these boys, and especially for men.

Pornography has been used as a weapon in war to weaken and demoralize the enemy's population. Is pornography the secret weapon of the feminist movement? By this decade, the 2020s, the feminist movement has grown in huge ways; it is perhaps the largest it has ever been. The use of pornography has never been greater.

THE MAIN DIFFERENCE BETWEEN HUMANS AND ANIMALS IS THAT PEOPLE HAVE THE ABILITY TO SEPARATE THEIR INSTINCT AND THEIR CONSCIOUS MINDS.

Men are hardwired to have sex, to reproduce. If you make sex readily available for a man, he will need tremendous willpower and strength to deny it, especially if he is attracted to the potential sex partner(s). With male animals, the nature is almost always to be dominant, to fuck, to reproduce, and the male will have no second thought about fucking the healthy female of his species nearest him. Also, if the male interprets signs of a healthy female of his species, but she is not, he will still make every effort to have sex with her, whatever his interpretation is, real or fake. The main difference between humans and animals is that people have the ability to separate their instinct and their conscious minds.

Sexual power has no morals, no conscious, no logic. Sexual power is instinct, decision, action. It cannot tell the difference between what is real and what is fake. Sexual power doesn't care.

Porn is fake sex, but obviously sexual power doesn't care: sex is sex, porn is sex, and it doesn't know the difference. Why go out on a date when you can have sex without going on a date? It is only man's conscious being that prefers a date. The availability of porn taps into a man's hardwired nature to have sex with what is attractive and right in front of him.

Most men who watch porn today have a very difficult time stopping themselves from continuing to do so. It's like denying food to a person who is starving. It is hard, not natural, to reject the influence of this power. Sex, or fake sex, becomes so available that you can have it any time, any place, day or night. If a high-sexed man is aroused and has the option to have sex without any consequences, he will. The only thing stopping him is the ability to control and redirect his sexual power by conscious choice.

Most men watch or have watched porn. A study was done that stated 82 percent of men admitted to using porn. Porn has not only wasted time and affected the way men think, it has also depleted them of their essential masculine and sexual power. To have sex or to masturbate: either takes an incredible amount of energy. This energy will seem to come from nowhere, and a man can have sex even when he is physically tired or exhausted. Ejaculation uses a massive amount of energy in one moment, and it depletes the man of this energy. After ejaculation men can continue to have sex, but the more they do the less intense and energetic the sex will be. Men can have sex until they no longer have an erection. After ejaculating many times a man's body will feel relaxed and calm, but give it a few hours or days and the man will feel aroused, energetic, and determined like before. The longer a man waits to ejaculate and use his sexual energy, the more aroused, energetic, and determined he will be. The man's sexual power needs time to recharge, and then the ejaculations will be much more intense.

The male ejaculation is the quickest and most inefficient way to express masculine sexual power. Ejaculation uses a great deal of sexual power in a short time span. After many male orgasms, the man needs to recharge, for he is depleted of sexual power and stamina.

During a male orgasm there are four hormones released in the body.

Oxytocin: also called the "love hormone," it induces connection, social bonding, and romantic attachment. Women have more oxytocin in the bloodstream than men, and it promotes uterine contractions for giving birth and also produces lactation for nursing. For men, oxytocin makes a man lose his erection after ejaculation, and this makes him relaxed and docile. A man also doesn't feel the intense arousal he did prior to the act.

Prolactin: promotes lactation (milk production) and breast tissue development. Women have more prolactin in their bloodstream than men. In men, prolactin can cause drowsiness after ejaculation. Also, high levels of prolactin in men can cause erectile disfunction and male breasts. It can also lower testosterone and dopamine levels.

Serotonin: this is your rest and digest hormone. This hormone promotes sleep and digestion. High levels of serotonin can decrease sex drive by decreasing libido.

Vasopressin: promotes proper cellular function. Vasopressin is higher during rest and lower during activity, causing drowsiness.

Male ejaculation releases hormones that change a male's behavior to make him more submissive and relaxed. Not only do the hormones change a man's state, they drain him of sexual energy. There will be a certain amount of time before the male returns to his original state of sexual energy. This could take a few days, weeks, or longer for the released hormones to lose their effect.

Take a highly sexed man filled with unstoppable passion and allow him to have multiple orgasms. This man may still have power, but that power is forced and does not come within him naturally. He is depleted of the primary source from which he was inspired.

Deplete a man of his sexual energy and he becomes easy to manage. He will be submissive and won't have a strong natural motive to object to or stand firm against wrong things.

As an experiment to understand the masculine strength of sexual power, take a cold shower without masturbation and then take one after masturbation. The latter will be much harder to endure the cold and stay motivated. You have given your power away and temporarily lost the vigor to fight. You can instantly notice your docile nature to connect and seek comfort rather than the assertive nature to achieve and endure.

> *"In today's world pornography is the mass castration*
> *of divine masculine power."*
> – STEFAN AARNIO

Four

How Does Porn Condition the Modern Man?

Porn has conditioned modern man to deplete him of sexual power on a regular basis: it keeps him from using his power and energy toward productive behavior.

Porn has conditioned men to obsess over lust and sex, causing them to further lose control of their ability to redirect their sexual power in a positive way.

Porn has conditioned men to become less ambitious by not only depleting themselves of sexual power, but also through making access to sex through porn too easy and available. When men aren't faced with challenges, they do not grow.

Porn has conditioned men toward dysfunctional relationships with women through the naturalization of the objectifying of women, through fake intimacy, and through not understanding real relationships.

Porn has consumed massive amounts of sexual power; wasted days, hours, and years of one's life at a time; and has caused depression, insanity, and more.

There is a tremendous amount of energy and time that is wasted on porn that could, instead, be put into something productive.

"When a man ejaculates, he expends tremendous energy—action-able energy, sexual energy, and divine, creative energy."
–Stefan Aarnio

Porn, in some ways, does not come by choice. It will find young men in our society.

The average age for a young male to start watching porn is 12. Boys are exposed to porn earlier and earlier. In most cases, porn will find them, not the other way around. Men are drawn to porn as though they are hardwired for it. Men are hardwired for real sex; however, their balls can't tell the difference, only their brains can.

Men make many failed attempts each day, through sheer willpower, to fight this urge. Unless you have unstoppable, never-exhausting willpower, you will always be fighting a losing battle. The will is weak and does not last. Most men don't want to continue to watch porn, and most men are ashamed after they have. This is normal. And it is a problem when we realize that today most men are enslaved by their sexual power.

Most men don't want to continue to watch porn, and most men are ashamed after they have. This is normal. And it is a problem when we realize that today most men are enslaved by their sexual power.

You might say that sex won't hurt anybody, but it will definitely hurt you. Sex always demands more. It never has enough. Even pornography is never enough. You desire a better high every time. It will get you into the wrong relationships, bad habits, and a disoriented mentality.

Our brains are hardwired for survival. A man's instinct is to eat, sleep, and have sex. Naturally, our bodies crave sex. If you weren't introduced to porn or sex as a child, sooner or later you might see someone, and you will think they are attractive in an arousing way. Sex is the most momentary pleasurable way to release a man's sexual power. No wonder men get hooked on it.

Video games highjack a male's sexual power. They are fake reality, and your sexual power doesn't know the difference. Video games create the illusion of facing challenges, achieving goals, competing, and making progress. Sexual power influences these behaviors, and this prompts males to play more video games than females. A study found that girls feel as competent as boys playing video games, but boys play more frequently because, for them, they increase the feelings of success and achievement.

Highly sexed males project what they see in movies and TV shows onto themselves. Watching challenges and successes can consume a male, for that is what they internally crave. A young boy will wish to be the superhero on TV, dressing up like one, acting like him, and wanting to change his name to the hero's name. Highly sexed men do this consciously or subconsciously when they rely on entertainment for their cravings of challenge, achievement, and competition. Men look to other men and aspire to be like them. Men crave masculine power and strength. The villain and the superhero both have masculine power; they are simply demonstrated in different ways. The status and power of these men are craved by the highly sexed because they demonstrate examples of what men are hardwired to do, which is to survive and procreate.

In 2022 $130 million was paid to one individual sports player for playing his sport. Sports have existed through much of history. Viewing a sports event has become much more available and accessible than ever with advertising, fast transportation, large stadiums, and the fact that you can watch a sport from anywhere in the world from your living room. Men have indulged in sports through watching them live and on TV, through fantasy sports, and with sports betting. Men will spend an afternoon fully engaged in a sports game. They want the feeling of competition and achievement, and that's just what they get. Men who don't—or even won't (if they could)—play on a sports team can be more passionate about how the team performs than players on the teams themselves. This is the passion that comes from their sexual core.

But sexual power can't tell whether you are the winner of the Super Bowl or a mere spectator.

Every time we use sexual power we are reinforced in the why and how that we did it. Video games, sports, and entertainment are conditioning males to use their sexual power in an unproductive way. They are conditioning males to prefer the illusion of challenge and not an actual challenge. The use of sexual power in this way decreases their need for real ambition, for the man is receiving fake achievement. Males are learning that their need to achieve can be filled with little effort. Why achieve something with a lot of effort when you can achieve something else with not much energy at all?

> WHY ACHIEVE SOMETHING WITH A LOT OF EFFORT WHEN YOU CAN ACHIEVE SOMETHING ELSE WITH NOT MUCH ENERGY AT ALL?

These shadow efforts fulfill men's instincts for survival in a fake way so they will be tame, submissive, and conform to authority in real life.

The twenty-first century is not the only time men's sexual power has been hijacked. Rome had rampant sex and entertainment known as the gladiator games. These were, in essence, the same as video games and pornography, just not quite as accessible and perhaps more or less artificial. Men were weakened, and Rome fell as a nation; this has been documented hundreds if not thousands of times.

For a highly sexed man, watching sports does the same thing as playing them. When a man does not sense challenge and achievement, he will crave it. Men have a need to use their sexual power. Porn, video games, and entertainment are way too easily accessible and, again, they will hijack one's sexual power if a man is not careful.

Why would you go out on dates if you could get "laid" for free by picking up your phone in your living room? And why do well in your business or compete in a physical sport when you can fill your needs for competition virtually? Men have the psychological need to procreate and expand. It's like hammering a nail into a piece of wood with no purpose of building anything other than to get a high from working. The male sexual power desires to produce more and do better. To deplete it in a false way programs men to continue to invest power into compounding a lack of productivity. Highly sexed men will always want more achievement and sex than before, whether that is in real life or in "virtual reality." If you achieve the goal of bench-pressing 200 pounds, it is no longer as fulfilling to bench-press the same 200 pounds. You naturally have the desire to bench more.

Meet the needs of a man's sexual power through fake sex and achievement and you control the very power which has the potential to build wonders and conquer nations.

DEPLETION

Depletion of this sexual energy becomes a great relief to highly sexed men. This sexual power, when charged, doesn't want to rest or take a break, for that is not in its nature. This is stress from the energy and the desire for sex. Men cannot just ignore it, so they develop productive or unproductive habits to redirect the stress. Pornograghy and video games are the most common ways of reducing sexual stress.

Constant depletion can be like taking antidepressants. You constantly need to replenish yourself, and the more you take them the more you rely on them. The benefit of an antidepressant is to take away the negative emotions that depress you. However, what is commonly seen is that people on antidepressants deprive themselves of positive emotions as well. Sexual stress should be dealt with; however, stress is essential for growth.

"TOXIC MASCULINITY"

The best way to attack your enemies is to turn them against each other. New ideas destroy old ideas and, perhaps, ideas that have worked in the past. The definitions of masculinity include attributes regarded as characteristic of men, including statements like "he's handsome, muscled, and driven; he's a prime example of masculinity."

The definition is indifferent; neither good nor bad. It could be bad attributes, good attributes, or both good and bad. Masculinity comes from male sexual power. Masculinity is sexual power, and sexual power is potential action.

Strength is neither good nor bad, aggression neither good or bad, and being driven neither good or bad. Strength, aggression, and being driven are not bad. The problem is these attributes are feared not because they are bad but because they have the *potential* for wrong behaviors and, naturally, humans greatly fear the potential bad more than they wish for the potential good.

STRENGTH IS NEITHER GOOD NOR BAD, AGGRESSION NEITHER GOOD OR BAD, AND BEING DRIVEN NEITHER GOOD OR BAD. STRENGTH, AGGRESSION, AND BEING DRIVEN ARE NOT BAD.

Women are turning against men and even turning men against themselves. The phrase "toxic masculinity" has been effectively pushed in the popular culture. It has wielded the power of fear in both men and women to focus on the negatives of masculinity and to disregard the positive need for it. Women try to set the standard for men, and most men drop to their knees to meet this standard. Again, in this case, these men have no control over their sexual power and, once more, women access it through men.

"Toxic masculinity" and "men should be more feminine" are attacks, not suggestions, even though they come across as being for the benefit of leveling the playing field for women.

"Toxic masculinity" and "men should be more feminine" are attacks, not suggestions, even though they come across as being for the benefit of leveling the playing field for women. Most women cannot compete in a physical fight with a man, so the woman resorts to manipulating her opponent with influence. Men fight with fists; women fight with words. The female uses sex as bait consciously, or subconsciously, and influences by creating "standards." If you meet those standards you may be given the bait. Which often is: sex. Even being baited by approval often doesn't directly lead to sex, but it creates the illusion and false belief that you deserve more sex. Most often this is the subconscious thought that runs through a man's brain: *If I'm nice, maybe she will like me.*

Many feminists support socialism and communism. One reason these women are against capitalism is not because they cannot compete with highly sexed men; it is because they do not have the same type of natural drive to compete with that which is in the core of highly sexed men. These women recognize the male sexual power and potential that these men have. They have seen or experienced it and have inflated the potential negatives this power can have rather than the positives. When one focuses on the evil of something, it can be very hard to uncover the positive need for it. So they resort to either bringing these men down or getting a portion of their power, and what it has created, especially if they are not a top sexual interest of these men. This is a power game, and not every woman can use a man's sexual power by either manipulating him or being a reflection of him or becoming a reflection of him by being his selected partner. The women who are not "qualified" to be a potential intimate partner with these highly sexed men don't give up there. They still do whatever it takes to bring them down by taking what their sexual power has created and turning others against them. The feminist movement, for many reasons, will frown on men who have strength, competitiveness, and success. A simple reason for this is because they cannot compete with the man's demonstration of sexual power.

Yes, women can have success, be strong, and be competitive. However, it is not in a woman's nature, necessarily, to do these things to the extent that this nature is in a man, and she does not have male sexual energy to fuel her stamina for these things.

Why do we need good men in our culture?

Essential masculinity.

Trying to turn men into women is like trying to pretend an aggressive pit bull is a neutered cat. At the core, you know that the pit bull is a pit bull, and a man still has sexual power, the nature of which is the polar opposite of a woman. You can try to delete it all you want, but there is sexual power within a man, and if you haven't found a way to redirect that power it will find a way to redirect itself.

The man may even be convinced that he must be docile, noncompetitive, and social. But the effort it will take to control this power without redirection will cause internal stress. Depression and even insanity can form due to the power within. It's something like how Superman didn't choose his superpower; men don't choose their sexual power. If this power isn't redirected, it will find a way to escape. You may fight and block it, but it will force its way, causing spiritual and mental strain to the point that it will break through in an uncontrollable way. This is the power of the male and sex.

You are supposed to be ambitious and have competitive energy. Pornography and video games rob men of this true power.

All men are by nature unsatisfied and looking to fill their themselves with things so they can be satisfied. But the human is not meant to be satisfied. We look for it, but it is never lasting; we look for happiness, but it is never sustainable. Men will realize that different things fulfill them in different ways. Some feel better than others. We want to choose the things that fulfill us the most, and mean the most to us, and will last. That is why men find purpose for these things. The things that fill men the most are when they are truly creating and giving to the world and to others. When they are giving to something other than themselves, to something bigger than themselves, that is when they find the most fulfillment. It comes when they love—not the love that is talked about in fairy tales—but when they actually love someone by giving freely to them without expecting anything in return.

Men are fulfilled by purpose. There is a purpose to sex, but what kind of sex? The high value man who spends his afternoon having sex with a harem of women is like the man who cashes in his investment early, only getting a small portion of the return rather than continuing to let his investment grow. While that man is wasting his energy and time, another high value man is being productive with his time and not depleting himself of his power.

The reality is the man who had sex with a harem of women won't matter. That sex was instant pleasure for long-term loss. A hook-up will not matter. You have nothing to show for it and gain only fake status. Men get hyped about and over-invest in getting laid; such a move, in reality, is of low value. High value doesn't waste, high value isn't free. If you'll have sex with any hot woman at the drop of a hat, what is the point? That you're free? This empowers the woman because she has control over you.

Sex without purpose is like hitting a nail into a two-by-four only because it was fun to pound the nail.

The purpose of your urges is to release, and by releasing itself it disregards what it is to truly love for another. The journey to overcome your urge is not only about succeeding, it is also about self-discovery.

True love is not a feeling, true love is a constructive action. It is about freely giving to somebody else with the pure truth and best of intentions.

Combine that with the feelings of love and attractiveness, and you have an unstoppable relationship.

CONDITIONING

Conditioning plays a big role in how this power is used. Conditioning also is another part that delivers an effect on how a culture functions with highly sexed men. Conditioning is anything that would influence the use or affect the masculine sexual power.

Animals are supposed to be aggressive and defend themselves. Though animals are a little different from humans, they are primitive like humans. Their instinct is to survive and populate. Some animals have unique roles in their gender; however, the usual roles are similar to the ones the human male and female naturally fill.

Why isn't my pet aggressive and protective? You can walk up to your pet and it would trust you with its life. Why do horses, cows, and sheep let you pet them on the farm? Meet one of these animals in the wild, and you will have an entirely different experience.

WHY DO HORSES, COWS, AND SHEEP LET YOU PET THEM ON THE FARM? MEET ONE OF THESE ANIMALS IN THE WILD, AND YOU WILL HAVE AN ENTIRELY DIFFERENT EXPERIENCE.

Human intervention has affected how animals respond today. Too many different types of training have conditioned animals in different ways. One conditioning that has been learned is helplessness. The animal is often unaware of its power, much like the elephant that is trained to believe that a tiny stake pegged into the ground will keep him from running away. Domestic elephants, as they are young, are tied to a rope that is attached to a stake. The young elephant will tug at the rope but never pull the stake from the ground. As an adult, the beast could easily remove the stake, but it simply does not because of what it has learned. Most of the time these animals are not abused; however, they are often in cages, surrounded by fences, and even some cages that will shock them and give them pain if they cross the fence. You control the environment so that they don't have to fight off predators or feel as though they need to escape. These animals don't know what it is to be free.

The second way of conditioning an animal is in teaching dependability. How do you train your dog? Animals are incentivized to do what you want; they are incentivized in two ways. One is with positive reinforcement. When your dog sits, you pet him and tell the dog it did a good job. The second is pleasure. You give your dog a treat when you call and it comes to you.

The third human intervention of conditioning is hormonal control. Most pets are neutered and cannot reproduce, and thus they don't produce the hormones that would enhance their ability to fight in a survival situation. One of the benefits of neutering your dog is that your dog is not as aggressive.

The second part to hormone control is genetics. There are many generations of domestic cattle that have led to the livestock that farmers own today; the genetics of this generation have been controlled. Even unintentionally controlled. All these animals were once wild and untamed. When these animals were first captured for domestic use they probably weren't the most cooperative beasts. Even animals that are taken from their mother at birth to be pets aren't perfectly cooperative, and I bet farmers would say they aren't perfectly cooperative in all farm-use situations. Naturally, however, the farmers will keep the calmer animals, and in breeding these animals this has an effect on their offspring. Now, if a farmer gets an aggressive animal that is uncooperative, the farmer is going to shoot the animal so it doesn't cause further damage. In this case the aggressive animals that would have first dibs on breeding in the wild would not get to breed and give strong, aggressive genes to their offspring.

I have nothing against the animal treatment I have just described so long as it isn't intentional abuse; the point here is that conditioning is real and effective. Looking at how children are raised, you may not agree with how some parents raise their children, but the job of a parent is to reward their child for positive behavior, scold them when they need to behave, and protect them from dangers in the outside world in much the same way a farmer puts a fence around his cattle. The difference is, unlike farm animals, your children become adults, leave home, and don't exist merely for the parents' profit. Your children will be sent out "into the wild," and if they are not prepared they will suffer and may even harm others.

CONDITIONING IN OUR CULTURE

The hope for these animals and children is that they have good and caring trainers/parents/teachers. Animals are trained young, and so are children. The most influence you can have on someone is when they are a child and their development is drastically influenced by their experiences. New conditioning is taking place in our culture. There may be a great deal of difference between animals and humans; however, there are some similarities in conditioning when young, and these things will affect their future.

Our culture is turning boys into girls. There is a conditioning of boys to despise their sexual power and deplete themselves of it. Public schools are made for girls. Girls do better in school and statistically get better grades than boys.

A boy's natural sexual energy is rejected and labeled as bad behavior. Most girls in school are viewed as saints compared

> OUR CULTURE IS TURNING BOYS INTO GIRLS. THERE IS A CONDITIONING OF BOYS TO DESPISE THEIR SEXUAL POWER AND DEPLETE THEMSELVES OF IT.

to boys. Girls do not have a natural masculine energy constantly gnawing at them to express itself.

Few people (especially in public schools) are forgiving of the boy who doesn't sit still in class, or who fights, teases, or questions authority. There is no proactive plan for these behaviors, only punishment and shame. The boy who rejects his natural urges to express these behaviors creates a recipe for self-destruction. Boys are taught to completely reject these behaviors in themselves and in other men, causing them to become victims of this "disease" rather than masters and reinventors of it.

Mixed-gender schools have affected boys by either intentionally or unintentionally comparing them to girls. When both genders are graded the same, it is hard not to compare. Also, while in the same setting it is hard not to compare behavior.

A boy's masculine instincts make it difficult for him to sit still and cooperate in a classroom. At least twice as many boys, compared to girls, are diagnosed with the disorder called ADHD. With ADHD, boys tend to show symptoms of impulsiveness and hyperactivity; girls tend to show symptoms of inactivity.

From a medically reviewed article, "Do ADHD Symptoms Differ in Boys and Girls?", the following were key findings:

Girls
- Low self-esteem
- Anxiety
- Academic underachievement
- Inattentiveness
- Needing extra help with homework
- Problems with executive functioning
- Trouble listening

Boys

- Impulsivity
- Overactive or aggressive behavior
- Difficulty sitting/staying still
- Talking excessively
- Interrupting others (conversations, activities, etc.)

You can see that boys tend to show ADHD in more of an active way, girls far more typically in a passive way.

In 2004 schools in Massachusetts, Maine, Maryland, New York, Virginia, Texas, and Utah started banning the game of dodgeball. Being competitive and physically strong in this game was seen as more of a destructive outcome than a possible good. More: schools have been taking words like *war* out of games. The vocabulary and phrases we have started using are very different.

In sex education the mentality taught is that you cannot control yourself, so you might as well have "non-consequential" sex. Most parents rely on the schools to talk about sex with their children. Obviously, they haven't been teaching abstinence. They also haven't been teaching regular depletion and uncontrolled sex; instead, these things are implied.

My gym teacher in middle school would tell me the drastic difference of boys' participation and athletic ability in gym class before the year 2000 and after 2000. Before about 2000, every boy would participate, every boy would be strong, and every boy would look forward to releasing his competitive energy in this teacher's gym class. Today boys are getting trophies for merely participating, and there are less opportunities to express authentic competitiveness.

School teachers and staff are taught to shun and punish bad behavior in boys. Is it bad behavior or is it natural behavior? "Boys will be boys" is a common phrase, right? Boys are growing and experiencing their masculine power for the first time. We forget the difference, and that this difference even exists. Society has been turned away from seeing the unique gifts of each gender. A person's gifts are neither good nor bad. Your gifts are potential, and you choose how to use them.

You cannot stop the potentially dangerous behavior of boys; seeking to do so will backfire. You have to adjust. Boys may learn to be "well-behaved and good students," but they will redirect their masculine energy into something else—again, often that is porn and video games. And, most often, they aren't watching soft porn or playing E-rated video games. The games are aggressive and violent. If they cannot express their masculinity in school, they will express it somewhere else.

AUTO-SUGGESTION

Society is verbally and formally teaching men to be like women, to deplete themselves of sexual energy, to be average, and to "not cause any trouble."

A person's brain is more greatly influenced by what one experiences than what we have been told.

Every time a man sees the cover of a magazine, an ad, or a Facebook post with a woman dressed immodestly it is a suggestion for sexual release.

The man's brain is hardwired to fuck what is attractive, not to use his sexual energy in a logical way. These things sell. They are hardwired into a male's brain. These magazines, TV shows, and Facebook posts get more views and more profit because of this simple fact.

Men are sexually triggered by visual cues. One body part or portion of exposed skin can completely redirect a male's focus and energy. The desire for sex goes from 0 to 100. This desire is distracting and can be incredibly compelling. The male cannot ignore the sexual stimulus. He can attempt to ignore it and may be able to control the influence for a time, but it is there and he feels it. The male's sexual power doesn't move him to think about relationship and intimacy; the male mind largely thinks about action and action only.

Women complain about how men view women as objects and how men "just want to have sex with us." An attractive, revealing female brings out the survival instinct and procreative behavior in a man. The interaction with a woman in a bikini and a woman in a modest dress isn't the same. The verbal interaction could be exactly the same, but the man's view of the two women will be entirely different. It's like placing a fat, juicy steak in front of a hungry lion. You're asking to look delicious. The woman may not be implying that she is asking for sex, but what she is wearing is.

SHE DOESN'T REVEAL HERSELF TO EVERYONE, AND SHE GAINS MORE RESPECT FOR IT.

Women who understand this either use immodesty to manipulate men or never reveal themselves to any man other than her husband. Men are more likely to respect modest women because such a woman's created impression isn't perceived as something just for use, but as an actual person and not just a commodity. She doesn't reveal herself to everyone, and she gains more respect for it.

The culture may not tell you what to do; however, it can greatly influence you. The wider culture can control your environment and what you see, hear, and digest. In history there have always been bans (thus, indoctrination) in cultures. Nazis burned books, and today there are bans on the media and the Internet. Social media tracks what you do to "personalize your feed for you." Music and songs by your favorite artists played while shopping in the mall are usually catchy enough to get you to memorize and sing them yourself regardless of whether the lyrics match your values. If you read the lyrics of most popular songs you hear many references to sex. More examples: most people shop for their food and go to their doctor for vaccines and medications. We don't know where these products come from, and we either take them because they are recommended or we take them because we are given an ultimatum: "take this or you may get sick and even die." But we don't know the complete effects of these products, whether they affect our brain, body, or reproductive organs.

Two more huge factors: social conformity and peer pressure. These are not always bad things; however, our brain wants to be part of a group and in sync with others. It feels easier to go along with a group whether it's to copy somebody else's work or just knowing what to wear in the morning. Our brains naturally desire to conform. You may have felt, at times, the feeling of being the outlier or excluded from a group. It is in this situation that you recognize the power of the group, that there is power in numbers. We desire to conform to groups whether that conformity is on social media, in church, or in some other outlet in your town. Whatever others in the group are doing or accepting, you are more likely to be inclined to agree with them. You do have the choice to disagree, and you may be part of another group that influences you to state that disagreement. In this case you are still conforming, just to the opposing group, and this will help you no longer feel like an outlier. However, without an opposing group you are likely to have a hard time being the outlier because of the nature of human conformity.

Your environment influences you, and the culture can control your environment. Today, regardless of how intentionally a man seeks to control it, culture has greatly affected him.

Five

High-Sexed Men Get in the Way of Tyrants

The high-sexed boy who questions his teacher is just like the man who questions his leaders. The nature of masculine sexual power is not to conform. It either creates or destroys. As long as there is sexual power left, men will persevere. This power doesn't look at things as others want them to be but as they actually *are*. Men who have high amounts of sexual power will either be your biggest ally or your biggest enemy.

Many fear male sexual power. We sense the change, or the damage—good or bad—it is capable of. We don't want to be overpowered by it, so when driven by it most reject it when really they should work alongside it. The high-sexed boy will naturally question authority and his teachers. If his leaders are driven by ego, the boy's questioning becomes an indirect attack; the leader's power is under "attack." His leaders become afraid of losing their importance. This questioning is an instinct of survival by testing the strength of his leaders. The fear-driven response is to shut down and threaten. This method wins temporary control but also makes an enemy. Nobody likes to be challenged, especially when they have much to lose.

Masculine men and feminine women look for internal strength. Internal strength is emotional control and self-reliance. Internal strength is the base of all strength. It doesn't matter if you carry the most lethal weapon if you cannot wield it and control it. Testing for internal strength is sometimes known as the "shit test." Women are not the only ones who shit test; men do it as well. Typically, a woman is known to subconsciously place this test on her man to find or confirm weakness in him. Women are attracted to strength. A weak man threatens a woman's survival. Men shit test other men, and also women. Men will tease other men until they react. This can be fun and silly, but it also confirms their reliability, especially when the shit hits the fan. Men also do this *subconsciously*. They dare their friends and challenge each other as a way of bonding. It's a way of testing each other's strength and making them stronger. It is men, especially, who bond by action and doing things together. Look at the unbreakable brotherhoods created in battle. Men don't have to speak to each other to bond. All they need is to witness strength and reliability through action.

The feminine mind doesn't easily bond the same way; however, it is attracted to this action. A woman doesn't want a man to tell her that he loves her; women want to be *shown*. They need someone to act and not reason with them. The soldier going into battle doesn't convince his wife why he's fighting; he just fights.

ACTION, AGGRESSION, AND SURVIVABILITY

Sexual power is inclined to break the rules, reveal truth, and even fight authority. This is to test strength and also compete with it. When high-sexed men sense a weak leader, it actually threatens their survival. They don't just want to act; they feel the *need* to act. "Hard times create strong men" is a long-held—and very true—phrase. High-sexed men thrive when they are fighting for survival.

> IF YOU WANT TO CONTROL A SOCIETY, CONTROL AND WEAKEN THE MEN. MASCULINE SEXUALITY IS POWER, AND THIS ENERGY NEEDS TO GO SOMEWHERE.

If you want to control a society, control and weaken the men. Masculine sexuality is power, and this energy needs to go somewhere. Productive or unproductive: it doesn't care. But the instrument will be affected by how it is used.

TYRANTS AND FEMINISTS ARE NOT AGAINST MEN . . .

Tyrants and feminists are against strong men. Masculine sexual power poses a threat to the weak and insecure. It is natural to attempt to tyrannically punish and control someone when afraid of them. Many women in today's society have a negative association with men. Most of these women have either had negative demonstrations of masculine sexual power or no positive demonstrations at all. Negative demonstrations of depleted masculine sexual power that women have experienced can take the forms of men neglecting them or neglecting their responsibilities. Also: displayed internal weaknesses subconsciously threaten a woman's safety and security. Negative demonstrations of misused masculine sexual power that women experience in men are abuse, anger, controlling behavior, and rape.

Women who've experienced these things have no trust in, and much fear of, men. Mistrust and fear of men drive women to seek to control and manipulate them, especially depleted men. The more depleted the man, the more likely the man will confirm to this depleted standard. Many times the negative will outshine the positive; unfortunately, that's just the way it is. This is not the fault of women but instead the misuse of the man's masculine sexual power. Any of these negative demonstrations of sexual power—like abuse, anger,

THIS IS ABOUT REDIRECTING YOUR SEXUAL POWER IN A PRODUCTIVE WAY.

rape, and lack of control—tells you much about a man's (lack of) internal strength.

So this is about redirecting your sexual power in a productive way. Masculine men shouldn't care about the affairs of feminism. Feminism exists because men are failing the shit tests. And make no mistake: you fail a shit test when you react to it. You pass one of these tests when you don't budge and are not affected by it but rather stay focused on what's important. In reality, women don't even have to shit test most of the time because men reveal their weaknesses before the woman needs to.

Feminism wouldn't exist if it didn't work. Men are conforming to and emotionally affected by feminism. Men shouldn't care. Bottom line: men are too distracted by the effects of the problem rather than the problem itself. Men are depleted of masculine sexual power right under their noses; they have no idea.

I am not saying controlling men is a clear, always-present intention of culture, and I am not saying it is not any intention at all. However, easy new ways of living, advanced technology, and times of peace (no war or threat of war) have made life much more manageable. Sex, entertainment, and having control sells—and most people are automatically drawn to these things.

Six

Without the Redirection of Masculine Sexual Power, Men Are Useless, Destructive, and Predictable

Sexual power wants to flow; that is its "goal," if you will. It flows by exerting its energy mentally, physically, and spiritually. Its nature is not to take into account the risks of how it expresses itself. That is why men naturally resort to expressing this energy in ways that are easy, even stimulating.

But there is a critical paradox. In order to redirect this power, you must first be able to say no to the impulse. This is where strength is needed: the strength to say no. People need and desire strength. People are attracted to this kind of strength. This strength is also known as *internal*

BUT THERE IS A CRITICAL PARADOX. IN ORDER TO REDIRECT THIS POWER, YOU MUST FIRST BE ABLE TO SAY NO TO THE IMPULSE.

strength. It fulfills the essential needs for security and safety, especially in people who are involved in your life. Without this strength, the power is predictably untrustworthy. Trusting leads to feeling secure. People look up to men and rely on men who are strong.

Strength gives you freedom to do with this power what you genuinely want. Internal strength is needed to break away from attachments, expectations, and influences. Cultural touchstones like society, family, and career all have the ability to enslave men in one form or another. Very often a man needs to rock the boat and redirect the aimless cycles in life. Internal strength will provide the most important power: the power over yourself and your circumstances. It is needed to say no when no is necessary. *Internal strength is free will in action.* It starts with combatting what is difficult, especially both the desire to deplete oneself and the *discomfort* of not depleting oneself of sexual power. Without strength all men will fall into an aimless, uncontrollable obsession with instant gratification, pleasure, and destruction. This is the nature of the flow of this energy. When strength is used to direct this flow of energy, it allows a man to pursue good and use the fearless source of this power to courageously move forward. Internal strength was used to fight the wars on slavery in the pursuit of freedom, both internally and externally.

People think power is in wealth, riches, status, and success. These things can be by-products of power, but the value lies in the *wielder* of the power, not in the result of it. The result can be a demonstration of the power, but that's never an accurate way to measure that power. You can have all the wealth and status in the world, but if you cannot control how you use it, you are truly powerless. Each highly sexed man has all the sexual power he needs, and if he cannot control the direction of his sexual power, he is also powerless over it.

The capability of this natural power is to create new leaders who blossom with ambitious and worthy goals, allowing these men to be motivated to solve complex problems. Men are much happier when they have deep, meaningful goals they try to accomplish instead of

THIS NATURAL POWER CAN BE REDIRECTED INTO BUILDING A BETTER WORLD AND DEFENDING THOSE WHO TRY TO TEAR IT DOWN.

being emptied by the successful achievement of shallow goals. A happy man has a great desire to feel important. This natural power can be redirected into building a better world and defending those who try to tear it down. Internal strength that has wielded sexual power for good has so much to offer a broken and unhappy society.

This reminds me of the movie *Fight Club* (which starred Brad Pitt and Edward Norton, 1999). There is a point where people of the city are trying to find the free men who are involved in the underground fight clubs. Little do they know how involved this redirected masculine power is in maintaining the city.

This great quote comes from that movie: "Look, the people you are after are the people you depend on. We cook your meals. We haul your trash. We connect your calls. We drive your ambulances. We guard you while you sleep. Do not f*** with us."

What makes highly sexed men unique is the ability to channel their energy and yet continue to produce and create without tiring. What makes them different is the instinct to produce what is deep within their core.

A feminine woman wants to be told no. She wants to trust you. She cannot trust your intentions if they are based on the fact that you like her and want to earn her favor so she will give you attention, affirmation, and sex. It's okay to desire these things, but never to change your decisions and goals because of them. All this means to her is that you are weak and untrustworthy, because when better attention, affirmation, and sex come along you will go running after those things. In this case your emotions make your decisions for you. It's like the woman who cheats on her boyfriend with another man. She cheats because her emotions like the other man more *in that moment*. Emotions change. If she breaks up with her boyfriend to be with this man, she is going to cheat on him at some point, just like she did with her now ex. Why? Because emotions change. Your morals and beliefs are much steadier. We all have some kind of morals and beliefs, but it is strength that allows us to stick to them.

People think they don't want strong men, but they actually respect them and even rely on them. People don't walk up to a lion and pet it because the lion has the potential to cause great harm. Men have great respect for the possible damage an unrestrained lion can do. *But they nonetheless greatly admire the lion.* Just like the lion, a highly sexed man won't always be loved, but he will be respected. And people in immediate danger will hide behind and support both the lion and the man for their protection.

Seven

Myth: "Women Control the Sex"

Women don't control the sex. Women merely take advantage of the rampant sexual power that men cannot control themselves. Men freely give themselves away as slaves of their sexual power. These men will find a way to release their sexual power through sex with their woman—or by other means. Men just want to release this power with a woman, and women will use this to their advantage. Men usually chase women because they think they are the prize. But men are not chasing women but chasing sexual release instead.

A man is not a slave to the woman he is in a relationship with; he is a slave to his impulses as well as a slave to actually being a slave. Let me explain. Slaves are told what to do. They don't choose; they take care of other people's responsibilities, and this keeps them from their own. Slavery, in this case, means no responsibility. Sometimes it seems as though it is easier to be a slave than to own up to your responsibilities. Men learn to obsess over the release and desire release, even consistent release. They will sell themselves to women to get reliable sex. These men desire the state of depletion. Why do men desire a depleted state? *They don't want the responsibility of controlling their sexual power.* Men don't want responsibility when it looks too hard; they cannot see the benefits of the responsibility. It takes effort to be a sexually charged man, in a state of sexual abundance, and not to jump at every opportunity to release all sexual power. It's like pulling back a bow and arrow and being ready to shoot. If you lose control you will miss your target, but you will also relax due to finally releasing the power behind the bow. If you wait and hold this loaded power without losing control, you can shoot it in its truest direction.

In the same way, it takes great effort to redirect this sexual power into something productive.

In the animal kingdom males and females compete for each other. Humans do the same. Humans aren't the only species who compete for a mate. Whoever has more options is treated as the prize. Females seem like they may have more male options. First, because women typically have less of an impulsive desire for sex than men, which means more men will want sex and desire sex with women who don't reciprocate their desire. Second, women generally have higher standards for men and look for men with a perceived higher status. (Refer back to *hypergamy* in chapter 2.) Men aren't as concerned with a woman's status when it comes to looking for a partner. Women typically have more boxes to check when it comes to finding a qualified partner. To men, she just has to look attractive to be desired. To the average male this limits his available options, while it give females all the options that she doesn't want anyway, but is there to settle for.

When competing, one has to go through two steps. One is to beat all the contenders, the second is to get approval of the prize. The prize gets to pick and choose. Be the prize and work on yourself, and you will be in a much better position.

When a man voluntarily abstains from sex he typically becomes moody. I call it a man's period. A man's birth control is safe sex, including porn and masturbation. Just like the female who has smaller periods after taking birth control pills, so is the man who is mentally and physically affected by frequent sexual release. Sexual release is an escape from reality and an escape from masculine tension.

Masculine tension is the state of being ready. It's something like your phone when it is between 60 and 90 percent charged; you are good to leave your house without charging it. Your phone will be ready when you need it, though it may well not be if you're only at 10 to 30 percent charged; your phone may be dead when you end up needing it. This masculine tension is like stored power ready to be directed. You are the master and commander of this power. A depleted man is likely a tired man. He will miss the opportunities when it matters and perform poorly. The depleted man is the man who could not give his all because he wasted it on something meaningless.

Many men live as though they must act a certain way to earn sex. Married men are told by their wives when they can and cannot have sex, something like a dog owner teasing their dog with a treat. This is not slavery directly from your wife; this is slavery to your sexual power. The man demonstrates weakness by having no sexual control. Women are not genuinely attracted to weakness. Toying with your sexual energy isn't only a test, it confirms to your woman that she doesn't want to have sex with you, a weak man. Most women do this subconsciously, teasing their man further and further to see how weak they are by seeing how much they can get away with.

It's something like a child breaking the house rules and looking to see how their parents react and if they can get away with more. A woman may also test her man, hoping he will pass the test so she can feel his strength and thus further her attraction for him, just like the child who gets in trouble to get attention from his parents, to feel their love and presence.

Women want you to desire them but don't want you to make them your top priority. They want you to be able to say no to them and prioritize your purpose. It is seen as the harder and more challenging path to prioritizing your purpose, and that is why men who say no to their woman and yes to their purpose are viewed as strong. The wife will plead with her husband not to fight for his country but will desire him more for his strength if he actually does so. It is the harder thing to do, but his love for her is not genuine if he is not true to himself and his mission.

Most women don't know or can't even begin to comprehend the effect their bodies have on men. Men are hardwired to notice an attractive female—just like when you're starving you're hardwired to salivate when you see food. The way modern women dress has drastically changed men's attitude toward women. Social media and immodest fashion are all over the place. Men can't hide or get away from this, and all it takes is one image to trigger a man's hardwired nature. Men who let such distractions control them show weakness, and women take advantage of this.

"The woman who understands [a man's] nature and tactfully caters to its need has no fear of competition from other women. Men may be 'giants' with indomitable willpower when dealing with other men, but they are easily managed by the women of their choice."
–Napoleon Hill, *Think and Grow Rich*

Eight

Abstain from Sex

Women are attracted to strength. Women are attracted to a man who can say no to his sexual urges and no to all women. The next relationship you are in, abstain from sex in that relationship and watch. The benefits in a romantic relationship from abstaining from sex are numerous. Women will go crazy for you!

Date them, spend time together, and kiss them like you normally would—just abstain from sex. You can do this. Put a strong boundary on it. This will show control in the relationship as well as control over yourself.

> THE BENEFITS IN A ROMANTIC RELATIONSHIP FROM ABSTAINING FROM SEX ARE NUMEROUS.

It is not easy—and that is one of the reasons it is so attractive.

Every time you demonstrate intimacy by kissing or touching and then stopping before it goes any further, you have just demonstrated strength. Your woman will get a high from this because every time you do this, you confirm her choice to see you, date you, or marry you. (She must continue to make that choice, if she wishes, even after you have abstained.) She wants to be with a strong man, and you are confirming your strength. She will test you and try to get you to have sex with her either because she has some disbelief in your internal strength and wants to make sure of it—or because she wants to reaffirm her attraction for you.

Women want to know that you are able to say no to them, and this is an extremely powerful way to demonstrate that.

Women don't want to lead. In our culture, many women have shifted into a masculine role, filling the need due to the lack of masculinity and leadership in society. (Women do this subconsciously as a way of survival. If a woman's husband dies and she has to take care of the family, she enters the masculine role, needing to be the leader to ensure survival for the family.) Our culture is a definition of figurative death. Men are dead in our culture, dead to their deepest identity as men. Many women have entered this masculine framework of living because of the poor demonstration of men in society today. Look at a woman operating in a masculine frame. She may fake it, but she is not happy. She is stressed; she needs support and reassurance. The feminism movement encourages these women, and they think they are doing the right thing. Women are encouraged to be strong, to be leaders, because they need to do so. Leadership and strength are not natural for a woman. The masculine frame isn't natural for a woman. A woman is happiest in her feminine essence, and she feels fulfilled when she is expressing her femininity. It is difficult to get a woman back into her feminine essence when she is stuck in a masculine frame due to a lack of masculinity. It feels unnatural. Masculine and feminine are opposites, and it is natural for humanity to find that balance through men or women, or both. Women want to be led, but they need someone strong to fill the role. Someone who will be more masculine than herself or the relationship will, most often, fall apart. You see this polarity difference in many relationships, both gay and straight.

CONTROL THE FRAME

Having "frame control" means you are controlling and leading the interaction. In a relationship to your benefit, your woman is deferring to you and entering your frame. Feminine women, when in a relationship with a man, want that man to be in his own frame. The masculine and feminine have different roles to play. A masculine man's role is to be the strength and leader in the relationship. Each sex has a role to play in the polarity of the relationship.

This is not about forcing someone into your frame; this is about maintaining your own frame. Your frame is the plans and boundaries you have for yourself, and where you want those plans to go. A man who stays in his frame is a man who has internal strength. It's easy to defer to someone else's frame, especially when you desire something of them—for example, sex. Having a frame is being able to make your own plan and lead. Deferring to someone else's, or a different, frame, looks weak because you are not the leader; you are not making the plans or decisions. Rather, you are deferring to someone else, hoping you will please them so they can give you what you desire. You can still maintain your frame when you defer to somebody else's plans. It is in the breaking of your own internal beliefs and boundaries that weakness is revealed.

This is about controlling your frame and not hers. Just controlling your frame doesn't force her, but it does let a woman freely step into yours. A feminine woman is happy to be in the frame of someone who is strong. The feminine doesn't want to lead or make plans. The feminine is unpredictable and emotional with a different purpose, one that is drawn to nurturing and creating the culture.

False frame in a relationship is when you are deferring from a place of need or fear. For example, let's take the crime of rape. Is rape controlling the frame? You may think rape is, but this is not controlling the frame. Rape is a frame; it should just not be your frame. Rape is one-sided, impulsive sex, usually because of lack of a man's sexual control. Rape is a man's sexual power controlling the frame, not the man.

Deciding to abstain from sex is allowing your woman to step into your frame. She is not being forced to have sex or not have sex. This is *your frame*, and if she is attracted to you, she will have to accept your boundary; therefore, to step into your frame. This will not deter her; she will tease and test your commitment to abstinence. Women will use a sexually active relationship to get her man to leave his frame and enter hers. She will abstain and say no to sex to get her man to defer to her and enter her frame (the myth that women control the sex). However, if you have already abstained from sex, she cannot control the sex because you already have.

IF SHE IS CONTROLLING THE FRAME, YOU START TO NEED HER MORE THAN SHE NEEDS YOU.

If you move into her home, you risk losing your frame, and she can much more easily control the frame. Every single, little thing can be used as an allusion to leverage power and control the frame. If she is controlling the frame, you start to need her more than she needs you. Therefore, she can threaten to take something, or herself, away, leaving you with the short end of the stick. You wouldn't want this to happen because it seems like an unfair negotiation. So you defer and further compensate for her wishes, therefore putting yourself in her frame. The more you defer to your woman's frame, the more you make it harder and harder to regain your own.

The possibility of her leaving seems extremely threatening if you are in a dependency mindset. Men who live in a woman's frame learn to become afraid of living in their own frame. If she leaves you, you will need to move out, will need to find a new home, will need your own household items, and so on.

On top of all this, the neediness and insecurities in a woman will reveal themselves very quickly when you are in your frame. Abstaining will naturally reveal each other's genuineness in the relationship. You can still find ways to use each other, but that becomes less likely and less often.

BUILD ANTICIPATION

"Attraction is not a choice."
—COREY WAYNE

A man may be afraid of abstaining from sex with his woman because he thinks she won't like him anymore and never have sex with him. Women don't need sex to be head over heels in love with you, and as long as you build the romantic attraction, she will still desire to have sex with you. *Women need anticipation.* Not having sex won't be the cause of her disliking you, but it can create the exact opposite. Women are emotional. When watching a movie most people don't just want to know "what happens in the end." They want to *experience* it; they want to see it for themselves. Just like abstaining from sex will keep your woman wondering what sex with you is like. More advice along these lines: when taking a woman out, don't tell her where you are going. Just tell her when and where to meet and what to wear. Women love to wonder about you and what you're going to do. They may ask and plead, but a woman in her feminine state will love to wonder about you and also what you're feeling for her.

"It's a scientific fact that women are more attracted to men whose feelings are unclear. Women like guys who are mysterious, interesting, and more difficult to figure out, and tend to lose interest in guys who are always available."
–COREY WAYNE

Most men want to "try before they buy," and thus want to have sex with a woman to see if they even like her. What a tragedy to finally marry a women and realize you don't like having sex with her! (This is the thinking, anyway, but it is flawed thinking.) One question for the men that have had sex with multiple women: was there any sex you had that was "bad sex"? Yes, some women are better at sex than others, but what is your goal for your romantic relationship? Is it to get married, raise a family, or just to have sex? If it's to just have sex, than good luck in an endless cycle of short-filled satisfaction with unproductive sexual depletion.

It turns out most men realize they want to get married and have a family; if not now, then later. Either way, I understand the desire to want good sex. A good place to start is to gauge your physical attractiveness to her and how well you connect during flirtation. You may not have sex, but you will definitely have a sense of what sex will be like, and if it would be good or bad. The amazing thing that happens when there is no sex in a relationship, besides the anticipation, tension, and strength, is that the relationship seems to blossom. It may seem like sex before has been a distraction and a waste of time. You will become creative with sharing intimacy, and the boundary on sex will bring about new ways or activities that become naturally more wholesome. You will become creative in finding things to do together that will make you learn about each other much faster than if sex were in the picture. Also, you both will be more focused on giving rather than focused on what pleasure you can get from each other. Lusting and sex can be a distraction from all the flags, good and bad, that you're looking for. Sex isn't everything; however, it shouldn't be completely disregarded either. (We will discuss this more later.) Many men have claimed that the best times in a relationship were when they decided to abstain. Just make sure when it happens it is your decision (as well) and not just hers.

The reason for sex at the start of a relationship is very similar to the reason to live together. You don't have to live together to figure out if this woman is a good fit for you. If some silly habit is a deal-breaker to you, then you're not attracted enough to that person to begin with. Everybody is going to have silly habits you don't like. (And guess what? You'll have them too.) Yes, you can still learn about them by asking questions and spending time together; however, living together has too many downsides for you as a man. Moving in with a woman gives her subconscious leverage in the relationship. She can have everything that a committed relationship offers without being in a committed relationship while having the freedom to leave without any real consequences. In one sense, that's a good deal! She may not own the home, you do, but this creates a new subconscious identity that makes her part of your home. Humans automatically create an identity for the things they are surrounded by, just as we naturally create hierarchy. This is how our brains compare and differentiate between things. For instance, children don't own their rooms; their parents provide them. Still, they all use the words "my room." Men should be the main giver in a relationship; however, do not give away your equity in a relationship. Giving should be reciprocated. But even with that expectation, even then, your primary focus should be to give freely without expectation. Give because that is who you are. Do not place the woman on a pedestal. This is not healthy for her, and in the end she won't respect it.

The more a women is involved in your life, the more access she has to controlling the frame. Even in a committed relationship, create and leave some space; participate in different activities and have different friends. Do not fear losing the frame in a relationship; just make sure you create your own frame. It's not only the woman who you want to control the frame with. It's your own sub-personality for which you need to control the frame. Plato said, "Love is a serious mental disease." Breaking up can be hard enough; don't make it harder on yourself than it has to be. You may see red flags and know that you should break up; many men do not. Every small obstacle in the way, like having to move her stuff out, or losing consistent sex, seems like a valid excuse to your sub-personality, and you will likely end up ignoring the red flags. Men are in a good position when they can break up with just a short conversation—and walk away with a clean slate.

It may seem like you are free to leave, but when you're in the relationship it looks better to stay with your partner than deal with the consequences of moving out and changing your lifestyle. Humans are programmed for habits, and sometimes we will do anything to not change our habits, even when we know it is bad for us.

Maintaining your frame isn't cruel to your woman; she won't appreciate you when you compromise. And as I said a bit earlier, women don't want to be put on a pedestal; they won't respect you as much if you do this.

Sex is a trap for your sub-personality. This personality is like your subconscious. It is not only when she moves in that she associates your home with her home but also your subconscious gets used to her being there. This associates, and creates an identity with, you and your home. The more sex you have with her the higher the likelihood of you becoming a prisoner of her sex. It doesn't seem like it is entirely you who is doing this. How many times have you found yourself in a situation where you say you shouldn't do something, but you end up doing it anyway? You will have internal conflict. This is what your sub-personality is. Your sexual power affects your sub-personality. The desire for your specific woman will grow, and she takes a place higher than other women because of the desire for sex. Again, do not make sex a negotiation. She did not give anything to you, and most importantly doesn't owe you anything. Nobody deserves that kind of worship other than God.

Yes, the divorce laws are against men in the Western world, and when married a woman can still divorce you, cheat, steal, and cause chaos in your marriage. However, you have more leverage than if you were not married, and now you have room to negotiate, unlike before. I'm not saying don't get married, and don't live together, but play your cards right and don't waste and lose your frame.

VET AND CONDITION

Vetting is like hiring or considering a partnership. You don't want to hire an employee and give them all the responsibilities right away. You want to take your time and look at your options, and this way, when you decide to sign legal documentation, you won't get screwed over if anything bad happens. But this isn't what we do with women. A sexual relationship will take a lot of sexual power. It's good to redirect sexual power into your relationship, just not all of it. When dating, you should redirect only a little bit, but not sexually. The man who puts all his money in a single investment is no man who is grounded or dependable. Invest a little into a lot of women, and the odds will be more in your favor. The man who stops hanging out with his friends and spending time in his hobbies has made an all-in investment. It's neither attractive nor productive. Watch the man who was crazy, ambitious, and daring with his friends calm down when in a relationship because he has given away all his sexual power. He has formed his life around a woman's life, and now she has leverage over his decisions and power. The power to choose for himself.

What's your goal? Maybe it is to date around for fun and intimacy. Maybe it is to get laid as much as possible. Maybe it is to get married and raise a family. And maybe you don't know. Choose a goal so you can put your time and sexual power to productive use. When you have a goal, you have higher value because your time is more valuable. Your time is a negotiation. It's either used toward your goal or away from it.

You are free to have all the sex you want; however, you are less attractive in the end, and sex does not serve you. Sex that was a day, week, or year ago is no longer giving you anything with a woman you are no longer with, and it has been a waste of an investment. You have nothing to gain from it. Momentary pleasure is just momentary; it has no value for you now. "Reliable sex" is a lie. You fill the "desire hole" that cannot be filled, and will always want more.

Even if you don't plan to get married, it is still okay to date around a little. Practice this while withholding your power. Men who have spent years dating around and depleting their power have wasted years of productivity. Do not go all in; take your time. Besides, women like men more when the man is not infatuated with them. Date little, or don't date at all, and redirect that desire for sex into an abundant life for yourself. Spend more time and energy on your other goals. Instead, build strong friendships that will last a lifetime rather than investing in a relationship that won't matter. Remember to celebrate your freedom by expressing your masculine power in the ways you choose, ways that actually build into your future.

If you are planning to get married, you should definitely implement more vetting into your dating life. Women want to be with a man who has options, or at least doesn't invest all his chips in one option. Don't get hung up on one woman. When you don't have the distraction and expectation of sex, it is much easier to not become blinded by sex and feelings. Find some good women. Take it slow and keep an arm's length. Men instinctively choose quickly, imagining the rest of their lives with a woman they have just met; women typically take things slow. It is easy to be flooded with strong emotions when attracted to a woman, but this will make you chase her away while also causing you to make illogical decisions—if you don't slow it down. You never truly learn about somebody from a couple of dates. To truly learn about another, it takes at least a year of dating without letting your emotions get carried away. Look for her good and bad qualities through her actions and not her words.

Have fun on dates, be creative, and make them inexpensive. Even if you can afford an expensive date, *you* are the prize, and your woman will have to earn that date. This gives you the opportunity to learn about her and leaves you no stress if the relationship does not work out. Your main goal is to build rapport. Have fun and don't take it too seriously. Never tell her that you have options; act like you have options. Do not chase her away with over-romanticizing. This will seem like you're seeking approval, or hold high expectations. This doesn't mean you cannot throw in a couple of romantic dates later on, but not in the beginning, and not over-obsessively.

As a man, both abstaining and being in your frame will definitely help filter out the toxic woman you date. First, most women without integrity who are stuck in a masculine mindset will quickly be deterred by you if you show them you will not tolerate being used or manipulated. Also, you will be able to clearly decide whether a woman is good for you through keeping your healthy distance from her. Why does it seem like other people can make better decisions for your life than you can? Because they aren't emotionally involved. A relationship built off of abstinence is much stronger logically, and you will not be as blinded from the emotional feeling that comes from sex.

While vetting, you are also conditioning your woman to respect you and your boundaries and to enter your frame. A successful relationship doesn't just spontaneously happen. Even if you feel as if you have perfect "chemistry" with your partner, there are differences and roles you will have to figure out. Couples subconsciously decide on roles in a relationship, and the polarity is constantly at work whether you both are neutral and play both the masculine and feminine roles, balancing things out that way, or one is more masculine and the other more feminine.

It is possible, but much harder, to switch roles in a relationship when roles have already been set. For example, if a man who was previously playing the feminine role and constantly in his woman's frame stops deferring to her frame and becomes his own strong masculine self, there will be conflict. Just like when the positive part of a magnet meets the positive part of another magnet: there is a repelling; both ends reject the connection. There will be a lot of butting heads as well as an unusual amount of testing from the woman in her masculine role, just to get her man out of his new masculine frame, and back into his feminine one, which has been making the relationship "doable." Men may attempt to change, but it is much harder, and they usually fail when doing this on their own. It is harder; however, it is possible, and it is encouraged.

From the beginning of the relationship choose to set firm boundaries and be the leader. Get your woman to enter your frame not because she has to but because she wants to.

You will not find the perfect woman. There is no such thing as "the one." There is no such thing as one perfect partner for everyone out there. This way of thinking is sometimes called *oneitis*.

This mentality looks very needy and weak. Some women are better than others. You can't find the perfect woman; you make the perfect woman. I have heard somewhere that artists say the best artists aren't the ones who just have natural talent or who train the most. The best artist has both natural talent and training. When vetting a woman you should choose a good woman, but you must also condition her to be a good partner.

For a committed long-term relationship, both you and your woman will change and will become attracted to other people. That is normal and okay, and yes, a woman's integrity should keep her from leaving you or disrespecting you. However, the relationship won't flourish if you as a man do not help and do your part by reinforcing her integrity for you by demonstrating internal strength and, thus, earning her respect.

SEXUAL TENSION

Sexual tension will build between you and your woman when you abstain from sex. This tension is a powerful feeling. The masculine and feminine are polar opposites, just like the negative and positive on a magnet. When you hold the magnets just far enough, you can feel the power of the magnetization. When you bring them closer you will feel even more power. The moment you release the magnets you no longer have that pulling sensation. This is just like the closer you get in a relationship without sexual release. After sexual ejaculation, both sexes will lose this tension. You both are no longer infatuated and not all over each other like before.

People desire something they cannot have, and once they attain it they are excited about it, but it wears off to where they want a new experience. Women will desire and be excited for sex to the point that the anticipation for it is more exciting than actually having it. Women will inflate the idea of having sex with you, and they may even tell you about this as well.

Abstaining from sex will demonstrate that you are a man of high value. You are a man who is earned and not free. You do not give your time, space, and sexual power away like nothing. These things all have value. You have become a rarity and are worth more. A woman is more attracted to a man with a purpose and a bigger goal than just his relationship with her. One reason women like romance novels so much is that they keep them on their toes in anticipation of what will happen, just like abstaining will automatically keep them on their toes because they know you haven't picked them yet, that you are vetting them. Just like the boss is vetting a new hire, so you are vetting a new woman. The boss demonstrates his value by having options and not needing you. So does a high-value man not need a woman for sex; he knows he is a catch and has other options. Be a strong man and have a strong position.

A healthy relationship is one that doesn't rely on or need the other person but complements and adds to that other person. Men who abstain from sex have a relationship that they can still develop effectively (even more effectively); they have no strings attached. People respect you more when you can walk away. Corey Wayne says, "The strongest negotiation position is to be able to walk away and mean it." You are able to hold your own and do not have a dependency on sex. Rollo Tomassi wrote, in *The Rational Male*, "In any relationship, the person with the most power is the one who needs the other the least." They can't take you for granted because, technically, you haven't chosen them yet, and women will realize this. Just like when you move in together, there are strings attached. You learn to rely on each other, and she can easily have less respect for you because she has more access to you. Yes, you can still walk away and even move all of her stuff out. But there are unnecessary obstacles. You want to both be free to leave. When you can leave, staying will be genuine.

Men fear that abstaining from sex when dating will cause women to walk away, but the opposite happens. Yes, maybe it will be a shock to her when she sees that you are not having sex with her or learns that you don't have sex until you are married. However, she will be more enticed by you and stimulated because . . . this is *different*. A woman's imagination is one of the best advantages men have in relationships. When she's wondering about you, she isn't thinking about her other options. Also, if she is wondering about you, she will typically become more fond of you. The imagination can be like another realm, another dimension. It has no limit.

Men may also fear that not having sex with their date isn't "alpha," or attractive, enough. Yes, women can definitely be turned off by men who are incapable of making a move and having sex due to a lack of strength and confidence. However, spontaneous sex can only be a shallow demonstration of strength, confidence, and domination. The big problem is spontaneous sex makes you miss out on so much more. You will still have to demonstrate strength and confidence, though in different ways. Demonstrate these qualities through the way you court her, by making plans and not taking anything personally. There is nothing in particular you have to go out and prove to her; instead, she will test you to see if you are weak. No healthy woman wants to be with a weak man. You can demonstrate true strength through not having sex with her, especially when she really wants you to. Power and strength is when you are able to have sex and don't.

If she leaves you because you didn't have sex with her, but instead remained strong and confident, then it was only a matter of low interest. She would have left you anyway, even if you were to have sex with her, or she is just with you to use you. Let's say she doesn't want to tolerate a sexless dating relationship. This is very unlikely, and nearly impossible, because to be promiscuous and to "value sex" to the point of rejecting abstinence is not a healthy grounded belief. Therefore, if she really likes you, she will conform to your beliefs and even be willing to disregard her own. If she genuinely values sexual encounters she will see the value in waiting for them. Someone who truly values something does not settle for the scraps of that something. Strength is the ability to say no even though it's easy and satisfying to say yes.

Sexual desire can increase or decrease for a variety of reasons; however this desire is not maintained by sexual practice. Sexual desire, and preference, is not a choice. Sexual desire only lives and acts in the moment, and time will not affect it. To abstain while dating will not affect your desire to have intimate sex in the future. You must cultivate the relationship and share intimacy—intimacy that can be shared in many ways other than sex.

Remember, this is not tyrannical or domineering. This is indirectly helping women give men what helps a relationship flourish—for both sexes. Rollo Tomassi writes, "Women are fundamentally incapable of loving a man in the way that a man expects to be loved by a woman." Men will crave for love, especially the unconditional love of their mothers. It is not natural for another woman to love you as your mother did. That love is for boys. And men are always unsatisfied by this love. Internally they are looking for the wrong thing when, instead, they should be looking for respect. Women are attracted to and want to respect their man. A weak, low-value man is very hard to respect. You as a man control the respect others will have for you, especially the women in your life. Make it easy to be respected, and a feminine woman will be grateful.

From 1 Peter 3:1 in the Bible: "Likewise, you wives should be subordinate to your husbands."

When doing this, women will test for insecurity. Past the test like you should, and she will see the strength and grow in attraction for you. Answer her test confidently and don't become emotional or needy.

What do you tell your woman when you're abstaining? First, don't bring it up for as long as possible—unless she asks you. You can either tell her right there, or tease her a few times, but do not overdo it. Advice: three teases max. Use it as an opportunity to be playful with her.

She may start to think: *Why doesn't he have sex with me?* This will cause mystery about you. This will leave her thinking about you more, which will increase her attraction for you. Usually a woman's first instinct is to think you have some insecurity, and that must be why you aren't having sex with her.

If a woman senses insecurity she will subconsciously sense weakness and begin to test. This is why it is super important to be ready for these tests. When she asks you, you need to tell her your reasons confidently, and no more. Do not explain in detail. Explaining in detail most of the time expresses uncertainty, and this shows weakness not because of what you explained but the fact you felt like you needed her to understand why. Over-explaining also may seem like approval-seeking behavior. Talk about it, but come from a place of what you think and believe and not just what she should think if she doesn't understand it. Women don't want to teach guys how to be a man. Women want you to already *know* how to be a man.

After telling her your reason(s), do not express emotion or approval-seeking behavior. Act confident, positive, and fun. Next, she may test you with her own tease, or a joke. Don't get upset or emotional about this. To pass the test just banter with her and act confident, positive, and have fun. View yourself as a man on a mission, one with a purpose, and take these teases as though they are not important.

Your woman will test you and continue to test you as long as you are together. A man is only a man in the moment. Anything good you have done in the past or will do in the future does not matter to her.

If you are dating someone who is religious, and it is assumed that they want to abstain from sex, then she may never ask you about it, so don't bring it up.

It's essential to tease, touch, kiss, go out on dates, and *yet* keep your space, and keep with all the dating fundamentals. Go for a "move" and keep going for moves. Doing these will keep the tension for sex alive. You always must keep the tension for sex alive. A relationship without the desire to have sex is a friendship. Without kissing, touching, and flirting you will end up in the friend zone, so you must make these other moves. You need to make it evident that you are into a woman *not by what you say but by what you do.* You are not bribing her, you are expressing sexual desire. Don't tell her that you love her; instead, you need to show her. Internal strength can only be demonstrated. Be confident and unbothered; just like in any relationship, you will have to maintain this demeanor. It's a little like this: blowing up a balloon to where there is a lot of tension, but not too much, to where it pops, or not too little, to where it deflates.

> YOU NEED TO MAKE IT EVIDENT THAT YOU ARE INTO A WOMAN *NOT BY WHAT YOU SAY BUT BY WHAT YOU DO.*

Many men have found it true that the best times in their relationship were when they decided to abstain.

WAITING UNTIL MARRIAGE TO HAVE SEX

Love is not a feeling; love is a doing.

Abstaining from sex before marriage creates a straightforward vetting process and places a clear goal in mind. Sex before marriage is like subconsciously saying "maybe." Maybe I want you, maybe I don't. I don't want to decide yet; I just want to enjoy you.

Barriers like birth control and condoms are subconsciously relaying skepticism. We want sex, but we don't want the result of sex, and we subconsciously relay that we don't want the result of sex with this exact person we are having sex with. We want the pleasure from sex and also the ability to walk away without any responsibility. We are taking from the other person the pleasure we have experienced—and nothing else. The message we are sending to each other is actually a message of distrust: "I don't know you," or "I don't want you to have my child, but I will have sex with you because I gain pleasure from it."

There is no love without trust. Not committing reinforces that you don't trust your partner, especially when you act like you are committed: living together and having sex. You are a man incapable of real love when you do not have standards. A man who lets an outsider in without proof of worth or skin in the game is not a man who can be trusted. A woman would first have to commit to you personally, publicly, and lawfully. Being your wife should be a place of high esteem if you hold to ensuring that you are a loving and trustable man.

Surely you've heard the saying "actions speak louder than words." Actions are stronger than words. If you want to read any person's true intentions, read their actions. What your actions are saying during a sexual relationship without full commitment is that "I do not trust you, but I will use you." Any barriers like condoms, birth control, or even pulling out confirm this statement. The barrier becomes a form of hesitation.

WITH HESITATION THERE IS NO LOVE

Sex is meant for creating new life, but what your action is saying is: "I'll take the sex without the new life." Every time you have sex with barriers you reinforce mistrust. Would you have sex if you had to completely trust your partner with the possibility of having a child together? Would they? Imagine how hurtful it would be for your partner to say no to having sex with you because you were ready and wanted to fully trust them with the possibility of having a child. What if they leave you because of this? Did they love you, or were they using you? And would they abstain and wait till they were ready? Actions do not lie.

Every time sex with hesitation (a placed barrier) happens it reinforces mistrust in the relationship. Every time sex with hesitation happens it reinforces mistrust in yourself as well. Your words are not in congruency with your actions. The likelihood of a person who has been through several sexual relationships like this, of carrying the baggage of distrust into the next relationship, is very high.

> THE LIKELIHOOD OF A PERSON WHO HAS BEEN THROUGH SEVERAL SEXUAL RELATIONSHIPS LIKE THIS, OF CARRYING THE BAGGAGE OF DISTRUST INTO THE NEXT RELATIONSHIP, IS VERY HIGH.

The beautiful thing about this is that whenever you're in a committed relationship that loves without hesitation, barriers, or boundaries, you reinforce trust in yourself and the relationship. Sex doesn't just become an activity, but an act of trust and love for each other. Your actions are saying, "I trust us with the outcome of our sexual experience."

You may say, "But I am giving the other person pleasure too." Yes you are; however, this pleasure serves them in no way. She has gained nothing of real value. It is a waste of time and sexual energy. This is not love; this is use. We borrow someone's body for pleasure. What is considered love has become a self-interested transaction. You may think you are doing her a favor by heading straight to sex with her, but you are doing so to please her because you enjoy seeing her in this way or want her to like you more, validate you, have more sex with you, and return the favor. As said before, it is like hitting a nail into a piece of wood just because it feels good. It has done nothing. Your biology thinks you are procreating, just like nailing a piece of wood with a hammer may make you think you're building something, when actually you are not.

When you make these choices, your partner actually becomes your victim. You cannot give this sex freely. You wouldn't have sex with just anyone. They have to be sexy and attractive. She probably doesn't see herself as a victim, and yet at the same time she may be turning you into her victim, one who uses you too. Does that make it equal? Does that make it right? It's like settling for scraps. They might taste good initially, but they will make you sick.

Sex without trust, and therefore love, becomes useless. Procreative sex is productive. It has the potential to become new life. Committed sex is also productive in the sense that you are not only creating new life but building a tangible bond with the person you are committed to. You are investing in your woman and life together.

Why invest in something that you're not going to keep? It's a waste of investment. Why not use your investment elsewhere?

Sex will waste not only time, energy, and focus, but the natural sexual power that can be redirected into something productive. To invest in a sexually active life that is not going toward a committed relationship is not beneficial for you, now or in the future. In short, it's a rip-off. You exchange sexual power for momentary pleasure.

The man who has been laid a thousand times has gained a little bit of self-esteem (in the moments) and yet has nothing to show for it. He has wasted years of time and sexual energy that he can never get back—and with women who are nowhere to be found.

Don't abstain out of shame or insecurity, but the desire to love.

KEEP SEX FROM YOUR WIFE
(AT THE RIGHT TIMES)

What about when you are married? Abstinence isn't just something you benefit from before you get married, but also after you get married. You should have sex with your wife, but you don't need to have sex with her all the time. There is a misconception that the more sex you have as a couple the better the relationship you'll have.

A study revealed that sexual frequency is no longer associated with well-being in a relationship when done more than once a week. Sex will help create a healthy relationship, but excessive sex will not make it better and may even keep the relationship from getting better.

The spark that was in the beginning of the relationship will go out in a long-term relationship unless you care for it. In order to do well in the game, you need to play the game.

Your woman never truly wants to be your first priority, but a close second. Putting your purpose first in your life will demonstrate internal strength, especially when you put it before sex. Sex should never become a habit as much as dates with your wife. This builds anticipation and excitement. Also, showing your presence and attention is way more important than sex is in making a relationship flourish.

Have you ever been without sex for a while with your woman, and then finally have sex with her? Sex usually becomes way more intense when you do this versus having sex on a regular basis. Abstaining will build on the desire to express your sexuality to your partner, and you will feel the stronger tension between the both of you. Don't just have sex in your marriage as a habit, but have it as a tool to spice up your relationship.

The person who receives a surprise gift is much more appreciative than the person who receives the expected gift on a birthday or Christmas. Don't do things out of obligation for your wife; do things out of the desire to give to your wife.

Also, don't make your wife always do things out of obligation. Help her do things out of genuine desire. Genuine desire isn't always there. It can be created. Create genuine desire by being wanted. A man of high value, internal strength, and full of mystery and ambition is desired. Never be or give in order to get—but because of who you are.

Bring back flirtation in a long-term relationship. Abstinence will help you master flirtation. The definition of flirtation is to behave as though attracted to or trying to attract someone, and yet for amusement rather than with serious intentions. Flirtation is an expression of attraction toward your partner who is not asking for anything in return. Subconsciously, a man's mind will act and flirt with the intention of being rewarded by approval, or sex, now or in the future. A man's subconscious primal desire is always there, spontaneously showing itself when unexpected. Most men subconsciously are unaware of their approval-seeking behavior. It is only when you become aware of it that you notice yourself doing things for sex or approval. When you abstain from sex, sex for you is not an option in that predetermined period, so it will help you express desire without trying to satisfy your sexual impulse. Sex can make you narrow-minded when interacting with your woman. What if you suddenly cannot have sex at all due to a physical reason? Would you act differently toward the woman in your life? Would anything change in how you approach her?

WHAT IF YOU SUDDENLY CANNOT HAVE SEX AT ALL DUE TO A PHYSICAL REASON? WOULD YOU ACT DIFFERENTLY TOWARD THE WOMAN IN YOUR LIFE?

Sex is more exciting when you wait, just like when you fast from something: it seems better than before. A man can lose desire for his wife because she is available and always the same as before. When you find yourself more attracted to other women, abstinence in your own relationship will help rekindle your desire for the woman in your life. You never genuinely desire your favorite chocolate when you have it every day, but when you haven't had it for some time your desire grows.

Do not deplete yourself entirely and over-indulge in sex with your wife. You can take some of that sexual energy and redirect it into other areas of your life.

DO NOT RUSH TO FINISH: THE IDEA OF SEMEN RETENTION

For a man, sex is a vulnerable act because he is entrusting his sexual power to someone to either amplify it or abuse it. If a man wants to be responsible and resourceful of his power, he must choose a worthy partner.

When having sex, there are a few things to keep in mind. You as a man can still demonstrate internal strength even though you are having sex. Demonstrating internal strength will make sex more enjoyable for both people involved. Sex should not be intended as merely a favor for each other to experience sexual pleasure; both partners should come from a place of genuine desire to give and receive such pleasure. It should never by forced or one-sided. This is why there is always value in foreplay. Either person may not desire to have sex when their partner does, so it is up to the other person to create the desire in their partner naturally and not through force. Use social queues and escalate if your partner is responding to foreplay. A couples' counselor, or you as a man, may try to make sex a negotiation, but that becomes non-genuine, obligatory sex even if it is consensual. Both partners must have the desire for sex. Without the desire it will have a negative impact in the relationship and cause feelings like resentment.

Naturally, a man can still desire sex with his wife even when he is upset with her; however, women don't respond quite the same way.

Men are much more likely to become aroused and desire sex than women are. If a man wants to have good sex, sex that is productive to the relationship, he will have to create the desire in his wife by maintaining his wife's attraction for him. As with most things in life, it is about working on yourself instead of changing the other person. If you want a great sex life you need to become desirable rather than trying to force your woman to desire you. You can gauge your wife's attractiveness for you through social queues. Truly enjoyable sex, to a healthy man, is sex that simultaneously satisfies the woman in his life as well.

A man who demonstrates internal strength during sex doesn't need—or want—to release his sexual power and ejaculate in a hurry. The ability to have internal strength arouses your woman even more, making the sexual experience that much better. During sex the strength is demonstrated in the ability to control the urge to rush to depletion. Subconsciously, she senses your ability to not succumb to her, or your desire, so quickly and uncontrollably. This is showing her you have the strength to say no by not giving in to her sexual gifts right away. This reveals to her that she does not have control over you. Men must always remember this: a feminine woman isn't aroused by a weak man she can control.

Make sex an experience. Women love stories and the anticipation of the story. Just as when abstaining from sex you build anticipation for sex, during sex you build the anticipation for ejaculation. A woman will desire her man to be in control of the sexual experience. Men are more likely to have control over the sexual encounter to the point that both partners usually wait for the man to have orgasm rather than the woman, and this happens for two reasons. First, the man may experience pain from epididymal hypertension—"blue balls"—when he does not ejaculate; and two, when the woman has an orgasm she can keep having sex—rather than, when a men has an orgasm, the sex is over because he becomes flaccid and will have to wait until he is past that state to continue. Men can either deplete themselves quickly or build the sexual tension and intensity, driving his woman wild with anticipation in the process. Make the sex last longer so you and your woman can enjoy more of the sexual experience.

The woman in your life doesn't want to know the end of the story right away, but instead to experience every second of it. She doesn't want to know when you will ejaculate. Your woman may tell you to ejaculate not only because she wants to genuinely please you, but it can also be used as a test to demonstrate your ability to say no to your woman in delaying your ejaculation, therefore confirming and raising her attraction for you. Preventing yourself from reaching climax right away will increase the sexual tension, making the sex encounter more exciting. Just like when abstaining from sex, you want to get your woman to the point in which she is the one who can't help herself in her desire to have sex with you. In sex, give her time to allow her to orgasm first if she wishes, indicating that she can submit to you and that she doesn't have to control her desires for you. Doing this allows her to relax and step out of the strong leader role.

> CREATE AROUSAL IN THE WOMAN IN YOUR LIFE THROUGH FLIRTATION, FOREPLAY, AND BANTER. ALLOW YOUR WOMAN TO STEP INTO THIS FRAME BECAUSE SHE *DESIRES* TO, NOT BECAUSE SHE FEELS OBLIGATED TO.

It's a man's job to control the sex. A woman's sexual desire is not like the man's impulsive desire. She needs to become aroused. Sex is not as intimate and enjoyable if only one person is mainly aroused. Create arousal in the woman in your life through flirtation, foreplay, and banter.

Allow your woman to step into this frame because she *desires* to, not because she feels obligated to.

With any functioning team, there are roles that are assigned. In a natural, healthy relationship, the man is the leader and the woman the follower. The couple needs to work together, just like in a dance. A feminine woman wants the man to be in control. Obviously, she wouldn't want him to be in control unless he was able to demonstrate strength and confidence. A man in his masculine state will naturally desire to play the leader role just as the feminine woman will naturally desire to play the follower role. The polarity of the masculine and feminine is a big part of the sexual attraction between a couple. The stronger the polarity, the better the attraction will be. The masculine naturally plays the dominant role as the feminine plays the submissive and passive role. The dominant role directly leads the interaction and is strong mentally and physically. The submissive role is happy to submit to the masculine. A feminine woman will be upset with a man who does not embrace his masculinity around her. You can see this especially when a man is seeking approval and enters a woman's frame by acting more feminine and delicate with her emotionally or physically. This behavior is repellant to feminine women, just like when two ends of a negative battery meet and reject each other. For men to maximize their attractiveness to feminine women, they must embrace their masculine behavior.

The purpose of a healthy masculine and feminine intimate relationship is to amply each other's strengths and attributes. The wise man will vet and choose a worthy woman to commit to him and amplify his sexual power rather than abuse it. The masculine role is to be the leader in a relationship by being strong and initiating. The feminine role is to freely express itself and dance along to the masculine lead.

Women like men more when they control their sexual urges.

WOMEN CAN SENSE SEXUAL POWER

Men who abstain from sex have noticed positive changes in attention and attraction that they receive from females. Pheromones are a chemical produced and released into the environment by an animal or human affecting the behavior or physiology of others of its species.

A woman may be very attracted to a man who is highly sexed because he may physically show attributes of a healthy man as well as expressing the characteristics of a highly sexed man. She may be able to smell the pheromones on him. People become attracted to what they perceive. Highly sexed men are perceived as having potential power, and this is alluring.

Expressed sexual power is attractive. A depleted man has trouble expressing his sexual power because he will never feel inclined to do so. Sexual power naturally will express itself and can be seen in many forms, including competitiveness, risk appetite, and confidence.

Feminine women want to be sexually desired, but they want a man to be able to control that desire. The desire has to be there first. A confident man in his masculine state is not ashamed of his desire, for he is confident and unapologetic when expressing it.

INDEPENDENCE

Take back the power that you may have lost from entering your woman's frame. I do not encourage walking away from a marriage, but I encourage being able to. Taking back your own frame can be as simple as learning how to go shopping and make your own lunches.

Dependency creates expectations and independence creates gratitude. If you know how to make your lunch and your wife does it for you, you are much more grateful. Instead, if she makes lunches for you because you just don't do it, and it becomes something you rely on your wife for, you will be dependent on her and less likely to be appreciative.

Have a life outside of her life. Make friends that aren't hers and start new hobbies she doesn't have. Become self-sufficient in as many areas as you can, if not all. A couple can complement each other without relying on each other. Long-term relationships can become dull because of sameness and too much certainty. Many of the good feelings that come in the beginning of a relationship are the feelings of missing and wondering about each other. To see someone every single day and know everything about them creates no excitement in a relationship.

All people need relationships, especially friendships. That is someone to talk to or share experiences with. You should talk and share experiences with the woman in your life, but she shouldn't be the only one, or then you have dependence on her, therefore giving her the power. When your woman can't spend time with you, you shouldn't defer to her plans and wait for her. Find your friends and hang out with them. This applies to fulfilling other needs as well. If you don't have a back-up plan for the things your wife does for you, that is an area in which you are depending on her.

If she offers to do things for you, gratefully accept them. However, do not rely on her, and make sure you continue to be capable without her. The goal in a productive, complementary relationship is to be giving and receiving from and with each other, but not to the point that it debilitates you from being capable yourself. You and the woman in your life should not be in a relationship to complete the other person, but to add to them.

You should be able to take care of your essential needs, especially financially and emotionally. To be able to walk away and never look back will demonstrate power. Always being able to walk away doesn't mean actually walking away. Sometimes you will have to when you're dating, but if she knows you can walk away she will respect and appreciate you more. Sometimes when you demonstrate power and walk away, she will chase you and enter your frame, and this in turn can improve the once-unsatisfied relationship.

Do not lose your frame to your woman, and do not lose your frame to the idea of marriage. Marriage makes people think they have to "sacrifice everything." Keep your independence. You need it so you can take full responsibility for yourself. You are much more effective when you help somebody after your needs are taken care of.

You shouldn't spend every moment together in a relationship. Couples often travel together, take vacations, and go on retreats together. Periodically, find a way to travel alone. Develop what I call your "independent mind." Couples, after being together, start to think like each other. They make decisions together, but often these decisions orbit around their partner's opinion.

Both partners should learn to be okay with each other's differences. They don't need to agree, but they will benefit by accepting their partner's differing opinions. We often instantly reject differences and try to make them the same or compromise in some way. Differences and opinions are not bad and still can be expressed, but there should be a boundary to where the opinions do not directly affect the decision you're making. It's important to differentiate the decisions that are made together and the decisions that are made separately. What you decide on the house and the kids are decisions made together—but not about what you or her are wearing or what you or her drive. Men will become dependent on their partner when making decisions because they feel the woman's opinion is a standard which must be approved, but in that case this leaves her with the power. You must maintain your independent mind and recognize your approval-seeking thoughts. Keep the decisions you make

> IF ANYBODY REALLY WANTS TO CHANGE ANOTHER IN A POSITIVE WAY, THEY MUST INSPIRE THEM AND NEVER MANIPULATE THEM.

together to a minimum. If anybody really wants to change another in a positive way, they must inspire them and never manipulate them.

You must maintain the boundary of the decisions you make together and the decisions you make separately. Developing your independent mind takes practice in deferring to your way of thinking and not somebody else's. A mature man is a man who chooses responsibility and is not chosen by responsibility.

It is natural for people to become dependent on patterns in their everyday life. Dependence is rarely ever a conscious choice. Break the pattern to make the relationship exciting, and work on your independent mind. Some occupations and careers help you unintentionally develop your independent mind by working extended periods of time away from home. Yes, sometimes it seems like a crazy amount of time to be away from your family and woman, but people often don't realize the gained benefit in their relationship. When a man is working away from home it is much harder for his woman to make his bed, fold his laundry, and make decisions for him. There is plenty of space for mystery and longing to grow, and this makes both people appreciate each other more.

A man focused on his personal purpose and mission will develop his independent mind automatically because his decisions will rely only on himself and the deeper meaning of his purpose.

Independence also teaches you to be fully present. A man must be present with whatever he does, whether that is with his woman or at his work. He shouldn't focus on his woman when at work, nor on his work when with his woman. When you aren't present in the moment you cheat your woman and your goals of your best.

Married or unmarried, you should learn to be alone. Many relationships start

> **LONELINESS ISN'T A BAD THING; THE OPPOSITE IS AN EXAMPLE OF USING YOUR PARTNER AND DEPENDING ON THEM. THIS IS NOT ATTRACTIVE OR HEALTHY.**

or remain together for no real reason other than the attempt to avoid loneliness. Loneliness isn't a bad thing; the opposite is an example of using your partner and depending on them. This is not attractive or healthy. In most cases when couples do this, it is reciprocated and both use the other to avoid loneliness. A relationship like this may last for a while, but it will not flourish. Depending on another person decreases your ability to give to them.

If single and not dating, soak in the loneliness. I highly recommending learning and developing your independent mind by being alone. You will learn how to do everything for yourself. Also, one of the most important things you can learn when going into a relationship is that you can be alone and be just fine. To know that you don't need another person gives you power. For single men this is not only an opportunity to develop yourself but to learn to redirect your sexual power into your purpose. Most single men waste days and years of sexual power in relationships when they could be investing that sexual power into something more.

There should be no rush to be in a relationship; there is so much value to be gained by learning how to thrive independently. Men become dependent on women as well as dependent on sex. Men act like the right woman, or women, will rescue them of the primal desire and solve the problem. This is deceiving and a misconception. A woman will seem like his savior; however, this is weak, and she doesn't want this part of a man in a relationship. Rethink your motives for a partner. If you are not able to be the strength in the relationship, both you and her will be disappointed.

The dependency is weakness. Needy sex isn't cool, it's unattractive. Neediness deters. Both men and women are surprised by and attracted to the man who ignores the hot women. Men and women can't help but respect the man who walks away from easy sex. To shamelessly like someone but not need them is the most attractive position you can have.

Master your sexual power before a committed relationship, and don't be drawn into one because of it. Men will automatically learn dependence, and they must retrain themselves from time to time to unlearn it. Spend a reasonable amount of time away from your woman, whether married or not. It is good to encourage your woman to make friends and invest in her own hobbies, if she hasn't already. Let her develop her independence. Genuine love is when you choose to spend time with someone even when you have the option to be somewhere else. Genuine love has no fences or walls; it is freedom that chooses to stay.

Last, it's in a man's best interest to have independence from sex entirely—both with his woman as well as any other form of sexual expression. A man's sexual desire doesn't have to be fulfilled through sex.

A man who chooses to be single when he has options is a courageous man. To do so will not only help your independence but mend your psychological wounds. Relationships can cover up and hide our deepest wounds until they can hide no more. Wounds can reveal themselves through neediness and "red flags"; however, healing must occur within you, and relationships can get in the way and seem to make things even worse. A relationship, and dependency, can seem like it is causing irritation to the wound, making it deeper than before. A man's relationships are never the problem; it is the relationship he has with himself. The relationships just reveal the symptoms of the wound.

To willingly choose a period of single life forces you to consciously and subconsciously work on the relationship you have with yourself. It is way more effective when you willingly choose a time to be single. The decision to seek and need a relationship reinforces the wounds.

A man in a relationship should thrive with and without his partner. That is strength. True strength will add to your woman, not use her.

Nine

Overcoming Your Sexual Impulse/Addiction

Most men, highly sexed or not, have masculine sexual power. They can choose to take up the responsibility of owning and redirecting it—or it will own and direct them.

Definition, once more: your sexual impulse is the powerful desire and urge you feel, typically, toward acting sexually.

A lot of men underestimate or don't even see the extensive power behind their impulse. It doesn't mean it isn't there. They haven't felt or encountered the power because they haven't tried to stand up against it, or, if they have, they haven't tried very hard. You cannot feel how strong the force is unless you counter it. These men are blindly being led and manipulated by their impulse, and they will never really understand the power unless they reject its leading with all their strength. In fact, nobody can personally understand or measure the true power of his opponent unless he has faced and beaten him.

"Only those who try to resist temptation know how strong it is. . . . We never find out the strength of the evil impulse inside us until we try to fight it. And Christ, because He was the only man who never

yielded to temptation, is also the only man who knows to the full what temptation means—the only complete realist."
–C.S. Lewis, *Mere Christianity*

The masculine sexual desire is a driving force natural to male human beings. Some people would argue that the desire is there to keep our species alive. Either way, it is there for men if they want it there or not. The male body releases hormones even before being born, and these affect the body and brain not just when these hormones are released but even during the absence of them. Men are born with this impulsive desire, and if there are no physical alterations they will have to learn to live with the full presence of this driving force. Some men may feel it more than others, but men will especially feel this power when aroused and sexually alert.

The use for this driving force has been misinterpreted through learning, development, and life experiences. During life all people are exposed to different things and occurrences that play an influential role on how we act and what we do. Every male with this urge will go through experiences in their life, but one of the biggest influential experiences they will have is the first time they are exposed to sex, directly or indirectly. This experience usually happens between the ages of 6 and 14. These boys do not understand the drive and power behind their desire, nor do they understand where it comes from or what they can do about it. In the twenty-first century sex talk has turned into a conversation encouraging sex as long as it is safe; however, most of the time the sex talk never happens. Boys will be drawn to sex, regardless, in time. Boys will learn how to consistently release this power through sexual expression. Masturbation and pornography become a learned, reliable source when a male needs to release the tension he feels from this force. Sure, there are downsides to fornicating just to fornicate, but these boys need to release their masculine sexual power. How else are they supposed to release the tension and power when they weren't taught how to release it any other way, or, better, taught any ways to harness it?

Maybe that boy was you. "A victim of sexual disease," or a discoverer of the quickest, most pleasurable way to release masculine sexual energy. Boys need to release their sexual impulse and don't know how else to release it. They find a consistent, reliable way to release their power through sexual expression. It becomes something that is learned and depended upon, and they continue this through childhood and into adulthood.

This sexual expression is the main method for dealing with a man's sexual tension; however, sexual expression on top of that can be a way of dealing with insecurities that can be experienced before or after your first sexual experience. Sometimes these insecurities come directly from a male's first sexual experience. To redirect your sexual power you should first identify the past insecurities. An insecurity can come from what is called a psychological wound, which is a past experience that has been interpreted in a certain way leading to shame or worthlessness.

The "cry for help" for your impulse is a real thing. It's when men have tried and consistently failed to free themselves from it. They have become aware of enslavement to sexual release and can't free themselves even if they try. The cry for help is a cry of hopelessness and last resort. They are in a moment of despair and don't know what else to do, who to turn to, or have simply lost any hope for freedom in the future. It is a desperate cry for some help or sign of hope to continue to bear this burden that is destroying the sense of freedom. They are ashamed, exhausted, desperate, and, most of all, feel alone. This can become the experience that makes them or continues to break them. Many men experience this moment every day, leading to shame and hopelessness. This cry is the call to change and becomes an insight into reality. You feel hopeless because your strategy to overcome your impulse is hopeless. You don't know where to go for help—or you do know where to find it but are too ashamed to go there. You either humble yourself and confidently accept the shame to look for the solution to your impulse without risking being exposed, and even put yourself out there . . . or you hold onto your pride and deceive yourself to believe you have the capability within you which disempowers you from acquiring the strength and tools available from outside sources.

> JUST LIKE ALCOHOL AND DRUGS, SEX IS ADDICTIVE. SEX CAN BE USED TO DISTRACT OURSELVES THROUGH FEELINGS OF PLEASURE AND BLISS AS A WAY DEALING WITH WOUNDS.

Before I cover redirecting your sexual power, we first need to uncover the deeper meaningful reason behind sexual expression besides the reason to release this seemingly uncontrollable power. Men will subconsciously act out sexually to seek validation or to cope with insecurities. Just like alcohol and drugs, sex is addictive. Sex can be used to distract ourselves through feelings of pleasure and bliss as a way dealing with wounds. Unlike alcohol or drugs, there is also a natural sexual force that desires to release itself.

Why do we seek self-destructive habits? It is not without reasons. There is a reason for all our actions. Not good reasons, but reasons. Why would we voluntarily abuse ourselves?

The reason men turn to habits like sex is because sex can be a temporary cure for feeling worthless. It will give you quick validation or numb you enough to distract you from the pain of feeling worthless. Men don't just impulsively masturbate for no reason. They will feel more inclined to do so when they are reminded of their worthless perception of themselves. Reminders can look like: having a bad day, or being rejected by a girl, a friend, and so forth. It's not the rejection that is causing men pain but the *meaning* they put on the rejection. It's not the idea of hating yourself but thinking you are never enough. People learn to define their worth by external circumstances. I am not saying that external circumstances do not matter, but to let them determine your value is a self-destructive mentality.

People survive off of feeling valued and important. It's one of our human needs. When men are unsure of their masculine value they grab their penis to reaffirm themselves. They feel valued, temporarily, for expressing their identity as a man through any form of sexual expression.

Sex will subconsciously validate a man when he is down. Men may have a need for validation because they can't, don't want to, or don't know what to do without, sex. Men will use sex to fulfill their need for importance as well as to hide the emotions that are behind their needs, like anger and resentment. When a man recovers from his sexual impulse, he will likely experience a new side of himself, revealing his true self, personal feelings, and attitudes (that he never saw before recovering). Still, he will need to work on his new self as well. Sex can be just a way of covering up and coping with emotional defects. Behind sexual drive there can be deep psychological reasons that get us to rely on constant sexual release.

> *"Deep inside we always knew there were other*
> *things wrong with us, and it turns out our addictions*
> *were really trying to keep us from facing them."*
> –*White Book*, Sexaholics Anonymous

Sometimes we think there is just a psychological wound that is keeping us from breaking our bad habit and impulses. Yes, a wound may be making things a little harder, but it is not just about healing the wound. To a certain degree, we all have wounds from the past that influence us to do things we don't want to be doing. It's extremely common to make excuses for yourself, especially like this one. You will think they are good excuses, but once you fully recover you will discover how much of an excuse it actually was. In the end we will have to find a place for our psychological wounds and needs as well as our impulsive needs. You can redirect your sexual energy just like how you need to find another way to heal from, or fill, your psychological needs in some other way. In general, you want to heal from wounds from the past; however, this will not stop you from succeeding in overcoming your impulse. But the healing will help.

The first thing to do is actively reflect and answer the questions that follow. The best way to do this is either by talking with someone or writing your answers down.

* * * * *

What psychological feelings are you seeking from sex?

What triggers you? Are you triggered during a certain experience?

What was your earliest memory of sex, and what could it have taught you about the meaning of sex?

Brainstorm any verbal, physical, or mental abuse you had as a child—intentional or not. What could this have taught you about your self-worth and where it comes from?

Do you feel ashamed by sex or masturbation? Why might this be?

* * * * *

Don't be afraid to spend your time with these questions in deep thought and self-reflection. These can give you understanding of where your shame and deep beliefs come from that can be making it more difficult to recover. This will also give you awareness of what feelings and triggers to look out for that get you to indulge in sex. Even just knowing and recognizing certain feelings and thoughts gives you the confidence and clarity to move past them without letting them dictate your habits.

You may find some deep subconscious beliefs to expose. Once you have identified any experience(s) and beliefs, you will want to spend some time reflecting on these. This can look like journaling more, and also talking about it with others. A hurtful, demeaning, or shameful experience is essentially a wound that will need healing which will come with acceptance and a new perspective. A wound is a sabotaging interpretation of an experience. Change the story you tell yourself, and put a positive spin on it. There isn't a magic trick to heal from these wounds; however, many people are surprised at the effects of even these simple mind exercises. It is not all about healing, but about transforming the wound and the way you see it. Obviously, you may have a different perspective now than you did when the wound happened, but what created the perspective was the viewpoint you had at the time. You don't need to change anything physically, but work on seeing these experiences differently in your mind.

Examples can look like teaching yourself that it is okay to no longer feel ashamed about years of masturbation and freedom to talk about it with a friend. Or changing your belief that love doesn't come from sex. Changing a belief is just acknowledging it and adding new perspective that makes sense to you. Spend as much time on this as you need. You may continue to find out more about your self-sabotaging beliefs as time goes on.

Remove all shame and self-judgment no matter how bad you think you are, because they don't help. Take your time with this; dig deeper into your answers. Continue to ask yourself why you felt a certain way about your experience. Discover if there are any other underlying causes.

If you find nothing from this exercise and think you should just move on, it can be beneficial to continue to go back to uncover more about yourself.

In addition, feeling worthless is something that many men may feel and experience now and from their past. It is not about comparing yourself to others but giving yourself innate value as a human being. It's hard to want things for yourself if you don't value or care for yourself. Most men give themselves this basic self-value conditionally, which is always being measured and questioned as to whether it is deserving. Self-worth can show up in taking care of yourself and saying no to things that aren't good for you. It is also addressed in putting importance on your wants and desires without judgment. This is something you can continually get better at by taking care of yourself and doing good things for yourself.

THIS IS A PHYSICAL, MENTAL, AND SPIRITUAL JOURNEY. BE READY TO GROW IN ALL THREE AREAS. IT LOOKS LIKE AN IMPOSSIBLE JOURNEY; HOWEVER, IT IS ACHIEVABLE.

This book is not about healing, but healing from past experiences and insecurities is a good thing for every person. Do not get hung up on what is a wound and what isn't a wound. It could make your insecurities deeper by going down a rabbit hole. The wounds are not the problem. It's the meaning we put behind them.

THIS IS NOT A CURSE

"With great power comes great responsibility."
—FROM THE *SPIDERMAN* FRANCHISE

Men have an impulsive sexual desire. If you don't have this desire, there is something wrong with your health. People will view this desire and see it as a disease or a problem. It is not. It is a gift that has been misused.

"As for you, what you intended against me for evil, God intended for good" (Genesis 50:20).

Welcome to the biggest journey of your manhood. To embark on this journey is not only to wield your biological gift but also to discover what sexual slavery has covered up and hidden from you. This is a physical, mental, and spiritual journey. Be ready to grow in all three areas. It looks like an impossible journey; however, it is achievable. Men have been where you are and have recovered from the mildest to the most severe slavery to their impulses. You name it, and men have done it. Men have expressed their power uncontrollably through prostitutes, molesting another, rape, and more, and have still recovered. You are no different, and your story is not unique.

This is the call to true empowerment. Power is nothing if it is not under control. It is only potential power.

The call to stop addictive sexual behavior could come to a man at any stage in his life. A true call is when a man decides that his impulsive sexual expression is no longer tolerable and negotiable. Many men experience the "desire to quit." Most men will already have the feeling of dissatisfaction of slavery toward their impulse. They will feel that the impulse doesn't come from a place of good intention but a need to release tension and fill an appetite. Most men will sense that something is just not right.

> *"The man who says he can, and the man*
> *who says he cannot . . . are both correct."*
> —Confucius

Men believe that their sexual impulse cannot be controlled. Why would they? They have never been told that it can. There probably hasn't been anyone, publicly or personally, demonstrate their ability to control and redirect their sexual energy. Why would men change when the only logical way to overcome their sexual energy is to directly fight it using their willpower—most likely without any moral support and encouragement. And if they do muscle their will to keep themselves from acting out sexually, then the question becomes: how long will he last? It's not like his impulse for sexual expression will go away. And so men fail. Without the encouragement and ever-consistent endurance, the feat to overcome looks impossible, and so the idea of it being impossible is reinforced in the man's brain. The man may try again and again because of the natural, unsatisfied feelings that come, but failing will furthermore reinforce the same belief that it is "impossible."

The alternative belief is to manage and portion his sexual impulse, and maybe he does so for a while, but the consistent forceful impulse will prevail against the willpower that seems like it has a limit and can only handle so much. What seems to be a socially acceptable way of sexual practice, like soft porn, turns into hard porn. Just like an addiction, the same dose never satisfies, and so the addict avidly seeks for bigger doses to relieve himself. The man who doesn't overcome acting out needs his "drug" more and more and in bigger and bigger doses. The man will start with casual masturbation or sex, which turns into pornography, than porn videography, then soft porn turns to hard porn. Hard porn turns into different varieties of sex and porn, keeps intensifying, and the man will find other outlets of sexual expression that are different, more intense, and more out of control. Keep going and the man may likely find himself someone he never imagined he'd be. He makes a line and keeps crossing it. You name it: prostitutes, massage parlors, cheating, rape, molesting, more. A healthy man's sexual desire will constantly nag him for more sex and better sex. This is the struggle of men. You can't have a controlled amount forever. That's not how it works. Lust doesn't work that way. Tolerance will increase.

"This will and should discourage many inquirers who admit to sexual obsession or compulsion but who simply want to control and enjoy it, much as the alcoholic would like to control and enjoy drinking."
–WHITE BOOK, SEXAHOLICS ANONYMOUS

The call for the man usually happens here. Where he has crossed an "uncrossable line" and has been given another chance or has faced the reality of his consequences—destruction of his family, his marriage, his finances, perhaps being in trouble with the law, and more. Most men wait until the moment of regret to change. These men look for the solution once more to finally change because, to them, their behavior just became, finally, no longer tolerable. The solution was there before; they just didn't see it. The mindset of "impossible" has been covering it the whole time.

"Every human being who reaches the age of
understanding of the purpose of money wishes for it.
Wishing will not bring riches. But desiring riches with a state
of mind that becomes an obsession, then planning definite ways
and means to acquire riches, and backing those plans with
persistence which does not recognize failure, will bring riches."
–NAPOLEON HILL, THINK AND GROW RICH

Don't wait for that day to come. Accept the call to the journey of manhood, the test of your real strength, and the challenge to grow into a powerful man. This isn't just a challenge but a true journey full of self-discovery, transformation, and experiencing your edge.

Your impulsive sexual slavery has covered up your true self. You will discover what you're capable of and find things about yourself you have never seen before.

They were there the entire time; you just couldn't get to them.

It may seem like you are taking this journey alone. However, other men just like you are on the same journey and are facing their own sexual impulses. You may share your journey with others, but only you can overcome your sexual impulse; no one else can do it for you. Most men ignore the call, but the ones who do so courageously fight for success. It takes courage to embark on a journey that looks impossible. All men have to confront and fight the battle against their sexual power. They either lose and become its bitch, or they put up a fight and make it their bitch.

This journey is the ultimate challenge for control, and the ultimate challenge for strength. Discomfort makes men strong; challenge makes men strong. A man's sexual urges are not supposed to be easy. If you cannot tame and control your power, it will tame and control you. Your power has to be constantly managed. This is a challenge, and this is uncomfortable, but it is there for men to become more. All men have the opportunity to prove to themselves and earn their power and respect, just as in the various cultures where there is a traditional rite-of-passage ceremony and initiation from boy to man. The boys in these cultures have to go through trials, prove their strength, and this usually involves excluding themselves from women. If they succeed they are accepted back into the culture—now as a man rather than a boy.

Just like any worthy journey, this journey will reveal treasure. Unknown treasure about yourself. And the count-

> JUST LIKE ANY WORTHY JOURNEY, THIS JOURNEY WILL REVEAL TREASURE. UNKNOWN TREASURE ABOUT YOURSELF. AND THE COUNTLESS BENEFITS AND REWARDS FROM OVERCOMING AND REDIRECTING YOUR SEXUAL POWER. YOU CANNOT MAKE A DIAMOND WITHOUT PRESSURE. IF YOU WANT TO GROW AS A MAN, THIS IS YOUR CHANCE.

less benefits and rewards from overcoming and redirecting your sexual power. You cannot make a diamond without pressure. If you want to grow as a man, this is your chance. Nobody has been able to enhance their life from nothing. It takes trials and experiences. Real life—and fiction stories—demonstrate this. Bruce Wayne wouldn't have become Batman unless he left Gotham, went to prison, and encountered Ra's al Ghul. Tony Robbins didn't become wealthy until he experienced financial rock bottom. The journey, and the challenge, is necessary. We attempt to look for the most impactful, life-changing experiences halfway across the world when they are literally right under our noses. This is your hero's journey, and this is where you will acquire your superpower.

The beginning of the journey looks straightforward, but just like any impactful journey, it never is. Self-castration is just a cover-up to the real you. It is the pacifier or the antidepressant for your emotions. You will feel more alive than before and will experience most of all your emotions, yet more amplified than before. You will feel your anger, joy, and other emotions in areas you have never experienced. Once you take off the lid to yourself you start to see underneath and everything inside. Most men deplete themselves to cover up the feelings and wounds they may be hiding, but it is necessary to reveal these in order to grow and embrace your manhood.

This is your call to manhood. Just as, throughout history, boys, in order to become strong men, were stripped from their mothers, in the same way you must strip yourself from pleasure and irresponsibility. Then you will face a worthy challenge and achieve it to be accepted back into the tribe. The only difference is that you must inspire your own journey toward manhood and do it without the assistance of your tribe or by creating your own tribe. Also, you do not do this for acceptance; you do this to magnify your strength. You do this because no matter what time period you are in, strength in a man is always respected, either by those who love you for it or those who fear you for it. All men are accepted today, but few are respected.

This is your rite of passage. Your journey that turns you into a man. A powerful man who has no control over his power is still a boy inside. The journey is about wielding power. Wielding the sword so you can fight the good battle.

It isn't your fault. This is what it is to be a man. The alternative to not taking ownership and responsibility for your sexual power is a destructive life full of emotions, like resentment and anger, that are never dealt with because you cover them up as soon as they show up. This destructive life is committed to self-sabotage and continual impairment in the name of one's own interests as well as leading to the consistent giving up of time and energy. Slavery to avoiding responsibility only gets worse, making you more reliant on your need to ejaculate—and possibly with a more arousing method—each time.

You either are progressing toward slavery to, or freedom from, your sexual urges. There is no middle ground. Your sexual urge is like someone else with a different agenda always fighting your ability to control it. If you aren't fighting being enslaved by your sexual urges, you will be enslaved by them little by little—until you have no control.

Don't wait to take action on your sexual impulse. If you wait until you hit rock bottom to do so, you will have wished you hadn't. Start now. It's just like a pile of dirt sitting in your room. It will keep getting bigger until you finally decide to clean it up. Every passing day you are losing your freedom and missing out on its numerous benefits.

It's up to you. If you deny the reality of this power, you will face the consequences of it.

Ten

The Decision

At first you may "feel" truly convicted, and that you have certainly made the decision to quit your impulsive behavior—but you have not. You only realize the lack of sincerity once you actually make the real decision to stop. The real decision is a must, a *nonnegotiable* on whether you will change your mind or not. It is a full commitment to the decision, an acknowledgment that you will feel the desire again and will, in the future, have a strong desire to change your mind. A great deal of the time the decision is driven by fear: fear that comes from the full realization of the consequences of your actions and your imagination playing out future consequences, driving you even more to fear the failure of your decision.

Don't just do this out of fear, do this for the betterment of yourself. Be encouraged by the countless benefits you will receive from this decision. You may be thinking that you have "ruined" your life, but it is *not* too late. The future looks dark, but in truth it has so much more that is unseen to you, in the moment, that it is yet to offer. This impulse will starve and blind you of hope, but it is there. There is more hope than you can imagine. This is not just about making your life normal. This is about enhancing your life and making it abundant. This is not just about fixing your relationship. This is about making the future of your relationship the best you have ever made it. It's easy to feel like there is just a mess to clean up, because that's all you are able to see, but the possibilities for a bright future are endless.

Again and again, the decision to quit will have to be made. Every time you are no longer driven by your sexual desire after the powerful release, you tend to make the decision to quit. Post-nut clarity will make you strongly feel the guilt and shame associated with your actions. The pain of these feelings will naturally encourage you to want to quit. You don't want to experience those feelings again, but the impulse becomes a seesaw. When you are driven with sexual energy, aggressively making you feel and desire the pleasure of sex, the feelings of shame and guilt are either gone or will seem farther from you than before. A man's sexual energy is that powerful: it encourages a man toward action and seeks to disregard any extra feelings that may be contradicting it. This power is just like when a man performs and does what he needs to do even when it is hard. Don't reject the power; embrace it.

In most scenarios, men make their decision to quit out of shame; the shame naturally encourages them to reject these powerful feelings. This shame develops into feelings of disgust, anger, and resentment toward their impulse. A decision made from feelings is a weak decision. Feelings change, and it is only a matter of time to where your desire for sex will outweigh your desire to prevent shame, anger, and resentment. These feelings cause a man to find the impulse unacceptable, and he will attempt to fight it. If it angers you, it will control you.

A DECISION MADE FROM FEELINGS IS A WEAK DECISION. FEELINGS CHANGE, AND IT IS ONLY A MATTER OF TIME TO WHERE YOUR DESIRE FOR SEX WILL OUTWEIGH YOUR DESIRE TO PREVENT SHAME, ANGER, AND RESENTMENT.

Men too often underestimate the power of their sexual desire. Your instinct is to fight it head-on by sheer willpower. Eventually you can no longer keep tirelessly fighting it, and once that happens you become seduced by your own impulse. Remember, men may be seduced by something external, but the root of this seduction is internal. Without their powerful desire, men wouldn't have to worry about external ways of being seduced. Most men will also use the pleasure of their impulse to cope with their feelings of shame and resentment, and this brings them to relapse again and again.

No wonder it has been found extremely difficult, and even "impossible" (as some term it) to control the impulse. The feelings created from making "a decision to quit" are based on feelings indirectly encouraging a man to relapse again. Shame—a normal feeling from relapsing—will naturally move a man to fight with his willpower, which will exhaust him in return, making him no longer able to fight, resulting in a relapse. On top of that he learns to cope with his shame and resentment by relapsing. Once he loses the feelings of being driven to battle against his impulse, the man relapses again, making himself shameful and resentful again, sometimes even more than before, getting him to fight the losing battle even harder. This a cycle that occurs based on emotional motives. Shame and resentment lead men to think they are preventing their impulse in the right way, but it is actually doing the opposite and causing them to relapse and become, once more, convicted by the feelings of shame and resentment to fight—and lose again.

The feelings of shame and resentment cause a man to reject ever accepting his impulse. The alternative to not accepting the impulse is to react to it and engage it. You will feel the full force of your impulsion when you are in battle with it. This is just like trying to put the positive side of a magnet together with another positive end. The closer you get to the other positive end, the more force you feel. Your impulse is stronger than you and has more stamina then you. Your impulse will win, eventually, every time, when you are facing it one on one.

You will not win the battle in a face-off. You stand no chance. The only way to win is to plan and strategize. If you know your enemy is better than you, you will naturally think to outsmart him, seek to gain an advantage over him, and avoid all possibilities of battling without some kind of plan.

Before you fight you first must know your opponent and what he is capable of. Forget what you thought of your impulse before. You must see it as it is—never less than it is. *To overcome your impulse you must first accept it and acknowledge its power.* You must understand that you are up against a relentless opponent that doesn't tire. Don't forget that this impulse is part of you, and neither anger or resentment will help you. You also must accept that you are a man, and this is what comes with being a man. Men are born powerful, regardless of choice. Feel and embrace the power, and you will be able to feel and understand the extraordinary power behind your impulse. To overcome your impulse, the decision to win has to be firm. Decide to fight it relentlessly.

Next accept that you need help, a plan, and a strategy to overcome your impulse. Nobody can win your battle for you, though others can help you. Last, accept that you cannot win on your own strength. The lesson is not to not fight, but to *not battle it yourself.* Nor is it to never use willpower, but to not use it to the extent that it is influenced by shame and resentment.

Once a man fully understands the power and the capability of his sexual power, he is aware of the slavery and manipulation it will have on him. Men will naturally fear this power. Do not fear it; learn to respect it. Fear will draw out emotion. Respect will allow you to think more logically and act accordingly.

When a man is overcome by his sexual desire and relapses, the common feelings are guilt and shame. Men quickly learn to fear guilt and shame. These feelings do not help the recovery because they are more destructive than constructive. They mainly bring you down rather than lift you up, just like negative criticism in a social circle has shown itself to be very effective in tearing a person down. After relapse a man should use the opportunity to be reminded of how real this power and influence is over him. Take a moment to understand the reality of your situation, to reinforce and upgrade your plan to overcome this power. Do not let shame or guilt creep in, in destructive ways, but use it constructively. It is not your fault that you are over-powered by this impulse. To believe it is your fault when dealing with most situations is never productive.

Decide to take this reality upon yourself to overcome and reap the benefits of freedom.

> FEAR FROM GUILT AND SHAME IS A DRIVING FORCE THAT CAN ASSIST YOU IN SUCCEEDING IF USED THE RIGHT WAY.

Fear from guilt and shame is a driving force that can assist you in succeeding if used the right way. However, fear is not a reliable force. You need respect and understanding when dealing with your impulse. This is how you avoid relapsing long-term. Start understanding and respecting your impulse now. People who consistently overcome their impulse take the necessary steps—almost out of awe and admiration for it. It is only after understanding its capability that men can see it this way.

Know your opponent and plan accordingly to win. Fearlessly make your decision to stand against your impulse—like fighting an enemy as well as befriending it like an ally. Build a relationship with the power and energy of your sexual impulse. You will learn to work together rather than fight each other. A relationship is not only between people but with concepts and objects as well. If you had a positive relationship with this part of yourself, it would be just like if you were to have a positive relationship with a mental disorder you have, such as anxiety, bipolarism, depression, etc. You are aware it is there and a living part of you. To overcome it you must work with it and not against it. Develop a relationship of respect not resentment. Learn about your impulse; understand it and its tendencies. Just as in a relationship, where your counterpart has needs to fill, and you are aware of them. Build respect and build trust.

Your sexual desire can communicate indirectly with you (just as a woman can in a relationship). This isn't a bad thing; this is just part of nature. Women often won't tell you what they want; they will indirectly tell you by behaving differently. You must learn the way of your impulse just as you learn the way of indirect communication. You will want to build rapport with your impulse, to understand it so you can live your life and use it to your advantage.

Most impulses men have today have similar tendencies; however, some will be different because of each unique person, their conditioning, and their experiences. This is your journey and your relationship. All are unique, and yet all have some similarities.

Your impulse is like a beast. If you were to face a beast head-on you wouldn't confront it lightly. You would magnify its aggression in yourself and then fight. You wouldn't be there only to win, but to stand up for yourself and earn its respect. Do not take this side of you lightly. You may not be an aggressive man on the outside, but you will learn to have the mentality of one. You don't always need to be aggressive, but you should have the capability to be aggressive.

STRONG, POWERFUL MEN AREN'T BORN, THEY'RE MADE.

Strong, powerful men aren't born, they're made. They start out as boys who form their desire to be like other men: forged through challenge, refined through the influence of strength, and enhanced through the demand and need for strength. Your sexual impulse is like a fierce dragon, a beast. It desires to overpower and devour you. It is in the way, and limiting you from accomplishing more. This is your challenge.

It's hard to believe a simple decision can help you change, but it can. To overcome your desire and make the truly convicted, nonnegotiable decision, you must believe it is possible. Maybe you don't know men who have overcome this. In the twenty-first century it has become more and more rare to find a man who is not enslaved by his impulsive desire. Most men won't share something that personal—if they are enslaved. If they are free they are much more likely to share because they understand and empathize with the journey toward freedom. All types of these men are out there. From the most enslaved to the least enslaved, but nonetheless enslaved, by their impulse. They exist.

The decision is more like a commitment and a pledge to overcome the impulse at all costs. The decision opens the mind to look for opportunities that will help. It wasn't as though the opportunities weren't there; they just weren't desired, or looked for, before the decision was made. When the impulse becomes a nonnegotiable, the distance to search for the answers and help is never a problem. It is about figuring out the solution to the impulse at all costs.

The decision for freedom is necessary but also difficult. Motivate yourself to make the decision. It's like you're dealing with two personalities: your impulsive side and your conscious side. Fill your conscious side with all the "whys," the reasons, you want to recover.

> *"People will do more to avoid pain than*
> *they will do to gain pleasure."*
> –Tony Robbins

To start, *find motivation through the pain of your impulse.* Will you find pain if the impulse ruins your relationship, keeps you from having the relationship you want, ruins your career, etc.? You already want to change; you just need to convince yourself to do the work to

YOU ALREADY WANT TO CHANGE; YOU JUST NEED TO CONVINCE YOURSELF TO DO THE WORK TO CHANGE.

change. Men want it to be taken away from them, but they also don't want to give it up.

Your decision needs to be about a 100 percent conviction toward change. If your impulse thinks there is a will, it will find a way. If you give your impulse an inch, it will take a mile. That is the way of your impulse: a fierce mentality that doesn't take no for an answer. The only way to overcome it is to maintain that same fierce mentality.

The decision to change can happen in a moment; however, there is almost always some type of journey to get to that decision. A journey of experience, knowledge, and beliefs that reinforce your conviction toward the decision. You must convince yourself. You are in the market and want to be sold the idea of quitting your impulsive behavior. All you must do is sell it to yourself. In the end, the decision is simple. However, you need to be your biggest supporter, and you need to be an unfailing source of encouragement to yourself.

Eleven

Sacrifice

"There is no such reality as something for nothing."
—Napoleon Hill, *Think and Grow Rich*

Nothing is for free. You must sacrifice something. The misconception is that if I just try hard enough to quit, my impulse will disappear. This requires not a trying mind but a willing mind. The difference is a "trying" mind is unsteady in belief and conviction. A willing mind is nonnegotiable and has the "whatever it takes" mentality. No, you won't lose your life in the process, but you must be willing to give it up to recover. You must be willing to sacrifice it.

> *"For whoever wants to save their life will lose it,*
> *but whoever loses their life for me will find it."*
> –Jesus (Matthew 16:25)

Sexual desire grows and inflates. The impulse for sexual pleasure becomes stronger and stronger. The man who is a slave to his impulse "needs it," longs for it, hungers for it. Many other pleasures in his life become dull compared to his ever-growing sexual desire. This man looks forward to it and doesn't realize that he begins to live for it by anticipating, with excitement, the next blissful experience he will have during his sexual release. The pleasure becomes his top priority, and his focus is drawn to it day after day. He has become not just addicted to the release, but to the feeling of release. A world without sexual stimulus, for him, looks somber and hopeless.

Great pleasures other than sexual desire exist for these men, but they are so numb because of their impulse that they cannot feel or see these possibilities. Sacrifice plays a big role in recovery; however, you also must be willing to sacrifice any present or future pleasure. You must be willing to give it up and go without it. It will not be taken from you. *You will have to take it from yourself.*

Men will want to keep around the occasional sexual pleasure, with control, just as an alcoholic will want to "control his addiction" by seeking to lower his use of, and yet still, drinking. Both learn that it doesn't work. This isn't how to overcome the power of your impulse. Its mentality is persistent, and to contain it you must starve it. Eliminate all sexually stimulating activities and objects. Your impulsive friend will eat them right up and guilt-trip you into more. You must fully sacrifice this pleasure. You can live without it, and you are better off without it. In order to recover, even married men will stop all forms of sexual activity, including having sex with their wife, for a period of time. When excluding all forms of sex, never set an end goal, just do it with the intent of continuing. Men will tend to not give it up but delay it. The fuel for this courageous period of delaying sex comes from the exciting anticipation of the pleasure at the end. What drives men to do this is the enhanced, moral, satisfying reward of achievement when they abstain; however, they are still hooked on the impulse because they are looking forward to it. Don't reward yourself with it or hope for it in the future. This will help you abstain for a short time but never for the long term. The need to fill the desire and impulse is strong. There is another way to deal with it, a better way.

EVEN JUST THE WILLINGNESS TO SACRIFICE GIVES YOU STRENGTH.

Even just the willingness to sacrifice gives you strength.

When experiencing shame and resentment from their impulse, men desire to give it up. After a few attempts they are usually smart enough to know that it takes at least some kind of motivated decision to abstain. Men usually never start this journey right away. They want to enjoy the last moments of their impulsive pleasure before they give it up. They act like the same desire they feel right now will turn off when they want it to. They will extend the deadline and extend it even more. To sexual pleasure-obsessed men, giving up their blissful feelings is so much to ask. They say, "I'll give this up when I'm in high school . . . I'll give this up when I'm in college . . . I'll give this up when I graduate." "I'll stop my lustful behavior when I have a girlfriend . . . I'll stop when I am married . . . I'll stop when I have my first child." The list of deadline changes goes on and on. "When should I start?" "Can I wait?"

We hope for it to change; we hope for our impulse to go away, or that some circumstance will magically make us change. Sorry to crush your dreams, but the only event that will help motivate you to change is the event you will regret: rock bottom because of your impulse. It's okay, gentlemen; it's normal. We want our impulse to be taken away from us rather than having to face it ourselves. To face it and take the journey toward freedom looks like a treacherous and lonely journey. Little do you know that your life actually is a treacherous and lonely journey; however, it is hard to see when blinded by your impulse. When is the right time to start? Now is the right time. The longer you wait, the harder it will be, and the bigger the mess will be. Don't expect to be rescued from your impulse, because you will be waiting your whole life.

Begin today. Right now. No matter where you are. If you gave into your impulse and ejaculated once, stop yourself there. Don't continue to dig your own grave. You already released a large amount of sexual energy. The tension in your body is not as strong as before, and the impulse to do it again is already less impulsive. The second you continue to attempt to ejaculate after the first time, you are no longer as motivated by the power you felt previously in your body, but you are still motivated by the pleasure of it. Men typically can't stop because they can't live with the impulsive energy and/or they are hooked on the pleasure from it. Men trying to recover will typically deplete themselves all the way and continually ejaculate several times so they can go a short period without feeling like they need to do this act again. This will work for a short time; however, if you are not able to live in a non-depleted state now, you will not be able to live in a non-depleted state later, and you will relapse. Not depleting yourself entirely can still be challenging, but also easier. You no longer feel the powerful "need" to ejaculate but rather, now, you just have the desire for it. It feels as though once you were unsuccessful at keeping yourself from ejaculating, you have failed, period, and to continue to stop yourself is pointless.

But to stop yourself is far from pointless. To stop yourself after "failure" can be challenging, but it will help you start to see what you are capable of. You practice resisting the urge and living with it. It reinforces your acceptance of the reality as well as your persistence to overcome it.

To play the long game will teach you how to succeed at the short game as well. The winning mentality with your impulse is all or nothing. Your all-or-nothing mentality is what will get you to the next step of recovery. Men feel like they must deplete themselves entirely; however, you don't use all of your sexual power during the first ejaculation, nor do you have to. Stopping yourself before complete depletion is a super helpful tool you should start using. You must learn to live without the need to experience sexual pleasure. This is an opportunity to break your attachment to it. Take advantage of the opportunity to strengthen yourself. Hold onto that remaining sexual energy, feel it, be aware of it, and don't react to it.

Stopping yourself after the first ejaculation is one of the best ways to train yourself to succeed when you are under massive amounts of sexual tension and desire to do it the next time. It is like lowering the weight on the curling machine to where you can actually curl it rather than just straining yourself and barely raisng it. You don't desire to pick the weight up, but you can, and you will get stronger because of it. You are not under the seemingly unbearable sexual tension you were under before the first release. See how long you can keep yourself from it. For an hour or two. A day or two. Or a week or two. Learn to go through your day with some sexual tension. This is where you can truly learn the nature of overcoming and living with your impulse. You will be always ready. There is no break. You will need no break.

SEE HOW LONG YOU CAN KEEP YOURSELF FROM IT. FOR AN HOUR OR TWO. A DAY OR TWO. OR A WEEK OR TWO. LEARN TO GO THROUGH YOUR DAY WITH SOME SEXUAL TENSION.

If you knew something terrible was going to happen the next time you acted out sexually, you would never do it. Sometimes you need a sacrifice in order to build that desire.

The measure of desire is determined by what you are willing to sacrifice. What is freedom from your impulsive behavior worth to you? How much are you willing to sacrifice for it? Nothing is free. What is the price you are willing to pay to purchase that freedom? The truth is you aren't going to get rid of your impulse without being willing to give up something for it. When I see men who want to shed their impulses but aren't willing to give up the needed things to do so, I know they will not overcome it unless they change their mind. A weak mentality will never overcome impulse. They don't desire it enough, and they are not going to overcome it without being willing to pay some price. Freedom isn't free, and anything worth doing is worth investing in.

The first and second month of recovering is always the hardest, and you will have to give up the most. Obviously, you have to give up the pleasure for sex; however, you may also have to give up many other things to recover. Men often value their sleep and won't give it up to recover. You must be willing to sacrifice sleep to get through the first breakthrough of recovery. You must be willing to give up your "adult pacifier." Be okay with feeling angry, cranky, or any other emotion that your impulse has been holding you back from. Work on them and resolve them as they come through, but don't be surprised when they come. You may argue and say, "Well, Daniel, I can't give up sleep. I need to be well rested for work or I can't focus and will get fired and won't be able to support my family and pay my sick child's medical bills." The list can go on and on. I do not argue against getting enough rest to work and perform well. However, this is the test for your true desire. It's all about the story you tell yourself. The story that says "I can't give up X, Y, and Z" because I need to support my family, or the story that says "I must give up X, Y, and Z" because I need to support my family, be a good role model, maximize my impact on my work and family life, etc. The ability to sacrifice something of value and importance to rescue yourself from your impulse will measure your desire and strength to succeed. To put those sacrifices into action will reinforce and enhance that desire and strength.

It's okay and normal to be distressed by giving up things you value, like sleep. You feel as though you "need it" and can't function without it; however, take action and do it because the nonnegotiable mind is a mind that sees no limits. A determined mind will figure out what to do and how to compromise. Be proactive in giving up your "needs." If I can't get a full night of sleep I will take a nap at lunch, I'll take a nap before the start of the day, or drink coffee, and/or take other steps. As men we are problem-solvers and are capable of handling obstacles.

To measure your desire, ask yourself: how much money is it worth to me to get rid of my impulse? Is it $1 or $100? What about $10,000? $100,000? Granted, everybody has a different importance and value they place on money, but if you place a decent value on your earnings, like most do, could you genuinely give up a "large portion" to overcome this state of slavery? If it would hurt to give that portion away in any other case, then you have created the desire to make the decision to succeed without negotiating.

In order to heal, this desire has to be a priority. It's easy to think of placing it as a to-do item later, but you won't overcome this never-ending impulse until you make it a priority.

You must also be willing to sacrifice your identity as well. Obviously, it is for the better; however, changing your identity can be hard to do. You must be able to rock the boat of your life. This is a transformation, and you cannot go through it without letting go of some things you identify with, like habits, desires, and relationships. It seems like in the end most don't need to sacrifice a lot, but they only succeed when they are willing to sacrifice.

What if you don't have the desire? Most men will not have it because of the illusion they have of the "pros" of slavery. This is, again, a normal feeling and mindset. All it means is that you must create the desire. You can create it in two basic ways: through changing your mind and thoughts about it, and by reinforcing your desire through action. How bad do you want this? An even better question is: how bad do you want to want this? Sometimes it seems easier to avoid the problem, and so we refuse to become aware of it. Most men know they want freedom, but the "want" is so small they ignore it. You can create the desire or want by feeding your mind the truth about your impulse, what it is doing to you, and what it is keeping you from. You can do this through reading, actively thinking, and allowing positive influences like people in your life who will relay the truth in what they say, but most importantly in how they live. Next is to learn more about your impulse and create a clear reason for overcoming it. This reason is your why. Why you want to succeed as well as why you don't want to fail. The difference is that one is motivated by desire and the other by fear, but they are both supporting reasons. Why you don't want to fail is usually the driving force and is much more powerful than what you desire by succeeding. This is the kick-starter to the whole journey, the fire under your butt. This is about what you fear and wish to avoid when living a destructive way. What are you afraid will happen? For example, my impulse will have a bigger appetite if I continue giving in to it, causing me to cross the line for myself with things like cheating, prostitutes, and more. I don't want to be a bad example for my children, break the law, or worsen my depression to the point of not turning back. It could be anything, and sometimes your reason will change—but you must have a reason. A reason for what you desire from this freedom and the fear of not gaining it. (Note: you can use fear as your primary reason because it is very motivating, but you should never let it be the primary reason in the long run.) For acting out of fear can become exhausting and crippling.

Sometimes you need to see and witness yourself taking massive action so you can start to place an importance on recovery. Act as though you desire freedom, and your feelings will follow. Become someone who is free, and mimic what free people do. Remove sex from your life as best you can, as well as any suggestions of sex. Use porn blockers, limit screen time; there are numerous other similar steps you can take. Take massive action to reinforce your desire by going to groups like Sexaholics Anonymous; pay for a program or a coach. Even go as far as physically destroying your porn device or even ending your sexual relationships.

You must *see yourself* doing these things, and the more you do so, the more your desire for freedom will naturally grow. Action reinforces the conviction of the mental

> YOU MUST *SEE YOURSELF* DOING THESE THINGS, AND THE MORE YOU DO SO, THE MORE YOUR DESIRE FOR FREEDOM WILL NATURALLY GROW.

decision you have already made. Use these techniques and start the recovery process even when you aren't ready, because the desire to recover will then begin to follow. No matter how long it takes, it's about the desire and the decision to fully commit. Strengthen that desire through action and mindset. Continue to search for help and the tools you can use. Take action; take massive action.

THE ACT OF TAKING RESPONSIBILITY FOR YOUR IMPULSE WILL INDIRECTLY HELP YOU TAKE RESPONSIBILITY FOR YOUR WHOLE LIFE.

Men don't realize the change in their behavior can be more drastic, often, than they know. This is what happens when you break a strongly embedded habit that has been unknowingly relied on to cope spiritually, mentally, and physically. No mere thought or feeling, no matter how strong, will change you. Action is stronger than words, thoughts, or feelings ever will be. You must experience transformation. Your impulse is covering you up from your authentic self. It's like the biggest layer, and once you start peeling it back you can clearly see what's underneath.

Freedom from your impulse will propel you into a whole new journey of life, allowing you to give more fully to the world. The act of taking responsibility for your impulse will indirectly help you take responsibility for your whole life. Your impulse connects to your life and to you as a man. This is a journey of understanding your nature more deeply and improving yourself so you can create an impact in your life, and in the people around you.

Twelve

The Advantage of Spirituality

You must acknowledge your failure and capability of failing in the future. Accept that you are imperfect. This doesn't mean identifying yourself as a "failure," but that, instead, what you have done before hasn't been working. Identifying as a failure can make you feel worthless and will slow you down. The stamina to be driven runs out when we don't value and deeply care about ourselves. It's much easier to care about taking care of yourself when you genuinely care about yourself. Don't let failing define you. Own it.

Many men, in order to recover, must have an ego death. Your pride and ego will get in the way of your ability to open your mind, limiting your awareness of knowing the nature of your impulse. Also, it will keep you from looking for other sources and tools that are necessary in helping you recover. The "I should be able to handle this on my own" mentality keeps you stuck. Not because you can't but because you limit yourself and may be beating yourself up with a made-up standard you have for yourself.

You may want to think and believe you can do it yourself and that you are capable of change. However, this leaves you vulnerable to fail. You become blind to your weaknesses. Understanding the truth that you are not perfect and will need help will only empower you. It will help open your eyes to what you really need and can make you stronger. Surrender your ego, for your ego will make you feel like you are making progress when you are just wasting time. To forget what you "think" will help you succeed. If what you and I thought actually worked, we would have succeeded already.

Humility will allow you to learn and grow so you can beat your impulse. The problem with the lack of awareness of sexually impulsive behavior in culture is that men subconsciously assume this is something all men know how to deal with and can recover from without any knowledge, awareness, or assistance. This is also why so many men are slaves to their impulsive sexual desires.

Recovery is not only extremely physical and mental, but spiritual. By "being spiritual," I mean acknowledging God, something higher than you. What this belief does is change your way of thinking to a way of surrender, trust, and hope. Many men get stuck in shame and the belief that they should be able to do it without help. This mindset can easily trap men into fighting an exhausting battle, and when losing and relapsing, the man will subconsciously doubt his own strength, making it harder for him in the future.

It can be extremely freeing and empowering to surrender yourself to God. To give him your impulse and all the pain that comes from it. You let go of your old self so you can find a new self. You can take a break from shame and beating yourself up. You accept yourself and everything with it. God does not scold you but accepts you. He already knows everything about you.

"Surrendering isn't giving up. It's giving access."
–Fr. Michael Schmitz

Surrendering opens a man's mind to opportunities that may help him. When his focus is narrow, the possibility of success looks scarce. The idea of surrendering is commonly used in addiction recovery, just as it is used in 12-step programs for addicts.

It's easier to surrender to something like God than just to life itself. God is someone you look to who has your best interest at heart, even if you don't know what that is. He has control. Instead of surrendering yourself to mere luck, you surrender yourself to control, God's control. Someone who has more control and power than you. This allows you to see both positive and negative experiences as opportunities that benefit you, no matter if they actually do or don't. Whatever you focus on will increase. With a caring God, we choose to interpret life differently. If it's a rainy day, you won't be distressed by the rain, but you'll see that it is a benefit to your lawn. Surrender provides stamina. It converts stress and worries into indifference and opportunity. Surrender can look like letting go of external things outside of your control, letting go of feelings of shame from your desires, thoughts, and the past. It can look a lot like optimistic acceptance.

As humans, we automatically try to make sense of things, but when you look to someone who is divinely perfect, the mental exhaustion and caution of making sense of things that are complex go away. We don't just get rid of our built-in survival mentality of making sense of things. We put this mentality into something more stable. God is someone we can't fully comprehend for the better. We seek understanding, and we want to know. It is important because if you make sense of your life, you are protecting yourself from likely forming a mentality of nonconviction and instability. People have a need to put their faith, trust, and identity in something. Put these into something that will not fail—in reality or even just conceptually.

Surrender takes the illusion of control away. Humans become overwhelmed with multiple tasks, decisions, and responsibilities. When we mentally give our problems to God with trust, we feel less burdened and are able to perform better. Putting high expectations on ourselves is draining and exhausting. It makes us weak for the hard tasks. The tasks and responsibilities don't go away with surrendering, but the expectations do. Without the stress and mental drainage of expectations, we do better, feel unwearied, and are mentally stronger. The impulsive man stops straining his mental strength and is rejuvenated to face his difficult challenges.

We become stronger when we connect with perfection itself. We understand our capabilities, and this gives more focus and life to our true capabilities. We face reality on a much greater level and are enlightened by the purpose we feel to serve something else, something higher. It's not only the spiritual help you will receive but the encouragement of having someone help you overcome your deep, dark secrets. Someone with whom there is no shame—because he already knows. Prayer is practiced within the self so it can be expressed outwardly. Every action starts with an idea that's given attention and focus in the mind.

TRUST

You have to learn to trust. It is scary stepping out into what looks like unfamiliar territory. Entering the unknown can cause men to second-guess themselves, become timid, or be abrupt. The unknown is a scary place for those unfamiliar with an ever-present sense of truth or God. Many life-changing journeys require you to step into the unknown, and men do not get through unless they hold onto a strong conviction (or belief) when there is likely to be adversity and uncertainty. God and truth are man's pillars to hold onto when the ground underneath becomes shaky. (The "ground" represents what they mentally relied on in this world.)

This was their sense of worldly things and where they looked for hope, love, and purpose. People naturally will hold onto things to find a sense of worth so they can persevere. It is only that man forgets that these worldly "pillars" to hold onto are never reliable. They will always change, and they will eventually perish. Only the spiritual is nonperishable. The spiritual can always be relied on, and it is always there. Most men only turn to the spiritual when it's the last pillar there, when all else has failed. One of our basic human needs is to have a sense of worth and belonging. This forms our identity, just as how food is necessary for life and affects a person's ability to be able to survive and persevere. People will need to find worth and belonging no matter what, but it is their choice whether to find it in worldly, perishable sources or nonperishable spiritual sources. A man is only as strong as the stability of his beliefs.

It's better to put your trust in God than luck. On a journey such as overcoming your impulses, you will lose conviction without trust. There are so many unknowns that can enter your journey that if you do not remain grounded in a reliable sense of truth, you can easily be taken off guard. When you are at war, you do not have the time or energy to question your truth or conviction, but only to relentlessly fight. You must trust the journey and trust the divine. You do not know what you will need to sacrifice or the result of those sacrifices in your life. The course of your journey will uncover certain things about yourself. There may be

YOU DO NOT KNOW WHAT YOU WILL NEED TO SACRIFICE OR THE RESULT OF THOSE SACRIFICES IN YOUR LIFE. THE COURSE OF YOUR JOURNEY WILL UNCOVER CERTAIN THINGS ABOUT YOURSELF.

an unexpected emergency that moves you to question your truth. The thoughts from your impulsive nature are not going to wait for you. Nobody can read the future or even conceive the possibilities of their recovery journey and future.

It's all about the mind. The mind can convict itself in any kind of direction with focus, imagination—and sometimes fear and desire. We must protect and guide the mind by having trust, and a stable trust at that. There are so many unknowns and possibilities that may happen during your journey that you need to have something to grab onto when all other things fail.

HOPE

Hope needs to be kindled and kept alive. You can find hope in God when all else looks hopeless. God is there when nobody else is, and he is your source of true stability. This stability allows you to be consistent. The truth is that men aren't usually afraid of the journey, but the inflamed passion for overcoming their impulse dies out very quickly. It is only through fueling the passion and having a stable source to do so that God brings the hope back and enlightens the journey. Suddenly, when all other sources of hope fail, God is still there. He gives you a reason to keep fighting and pursuing the truth for yourself. With God there is meaning in your life and a reason for hope to be alive. All else will perish in this life, but God will be there, and your actions and intentions will count for something.

Your goal is no longer worthless, but means so much more. Through God you can build the needed hope to recover. Without hope, men are not able to persist against their impulses. Hope is the fuel that drives you forward, surpassing obstacles and fear. Hope is the fuel of the will to give it more strength and to stretch itself. Without hope, we do not have a vision for the future and the journey that will help us take the next necessary steps. You need trust and surrender, but it is not your driving force. Hope quickens your recovery and is the excitement and passion behind the journey. It is your motivation and inspiration.

To believe in God is to believe in possibility. You need to encourage your belief of success in and along the journey. God is there, but it is up to us to connect with him. We do much better if we are working together. (Even the illusion of working beside someone can lift a person's spirits.) Remind yourself that the all-powerful God has a plan for you. Let God focus on the details so you can focus on the execution. Put your worries and concerns in his hands. Build a vision and work side by side with someone who may have an even better vision for yourself.

PRAYER

Prayer is our way of communicating with God. The rewards we receive from prayer and the acknowledgment of God are not just spiritual but also provide rewards through our actions. The act of praying is a powerful tool. Every time you pray you have to humble yourself because you either are conversing with someone more powerful than you or asking for help. Prayer teaches you humility. Prayer is an indirect practice of humility. Humility is the opposite of pride, which is the vice that can prevent men from truly stretching themselves to become more. Humility will free you from the limitations of pride. In order to succeed in life, in this journey, you must continually learn, adapt, and grow. Pride is a vice that can be reduced, but it will never die. Only practice and persistence will keep it at bay.

Praying also takes the form of sacrifice by the giving up of your time and attention so you can pray. As I mentioned previously, the willingness to sacrifice what you have correlates with the amount of desire to succeed.

What you pray about, you focus on and think about. This brings out the problem through your undivided attention, which enlightens the imagination to plan and solve. Humans often think in solution-based ways, especially men. Once you bring things into the light a man's instinct is to solve and accomplish. This is part of the gift men have. What the practice of prayer does as well is *remind* and *prioritize*. The human brain is often sidetracked, but the habit of prayer helps us remember what's important and what we should be focused on.

Prayer is often an act of intentional surrender by mentally giving your problems away to someone who can take the control that you don't have over those problems. Our possessive brains need to learn what to *not* identify with. Humans live by identity and will automatically identify with things that can cause good as well as turmoil. This is why minimalism is so sought after by many. It is freedom from an overbearing amount of things we identify with, just like how our physical storage seems to have some hold, some capacity on our brains. The more we own, the more anxiety we have about the things we own. When we clean and get rid of things, it is a freeing experience. We often over-identify with our problems, getting lost in the details, causing us to trip up and forget the point of the mission. The mental identity brings along with it some kind of inherent responsibility. This new identity becomes an overbearing liability, decreasing our performance. You can give away your storage and get rid of some of your physical identity, and you can also give away your mental identity through prayer to God. Surrender to God in prayer. Ask him to receive your impulses. The next impulse will still exist, but surren-

THE MORE WE OWN, THE MORE ANXIETY WE HAVE ABOUT THE THINGS WE OWN. WHEN WE CLEAN AND GET RID OF THINGS, IT IS A FREEING EXPERIENCE.

der eases your mental burden. Just like getting rid of your storage: it is not on your mind and you don't identify with it anymore.

The more you connect with God, the more you will associate yourself with his stability and naturally feel more confident in finding surrender, trust, and hope in him. This is the same way your identity today did not become this way overnight. People are mostly unaware of the formation of their identity, but it is formed through choice and focus that is mostly formed in the subconscious. What you see and experience influences what you think you should identify with, whether that is a relationship, career, sport, role model, way of life, fear, or desire. You can change your identity by changing your focus and choices. This usually takes time and consistency.

You may be able to quickly alter and change your lifestyle, but naturally this new identity will be shallowly rooted. It is only through continuous focus and conscious choosing that the roots of your identity will grow. Going back to uplift those roots from past wounds and desires will help the process as well. Identifying with anything is as simple as creating a relationship or association with it. Just as how true relationships need time spent together, as well as focus, attention, and experiences, so does creating an identity with God. Prayer is time, focus, and attention with God. Your awareness of God and how present you let him be in your life will help create experiences that will increase that stable identity. A relationship with the divine will give you strength. It will make you less reliant on worldly, unstable identities and free you from those expectations. With God you will never be alone.

God is usually the last resort—and yet the easiest one. You can approach him in any way, angry or happy, and he will not react. You can approach him with sincere honesty, without seeking approval, because he knows you better than you know yourself. He is accessible anytime, anywhere, and will always be there to listen to you. God, to you, is only as good as you make your relationship with him.

The alternative to not developing a relationship with God or anything spiritual is that your identity is fragile. You may have a strong belief in your ability to achieve your goal; however, when your identity breaks, your strong belief is likely to be affected as well. Without the gifts that a relationship with God will supply, you can anticipate roadblocks along the way and inconsistent levels of conviction. You will be more likely to disregard the opportunities to grow and be filled with a burdensome pressure on yourself and your anxiety, making it too exhausting to persevere when perseverance is just what is needed.

In an ever-changing and perishing world that has *some* good but always so much hardship, you will most likely question yourself and your goals and lose hope and vision of the future.

Last is this benefit: God helps remove our shame. To heal our wounds and feelings of shame takes attention, and it takes time. God is usually that important first step. He already knows you, and you can speak to him in silence. Confessing to him gets you ready to confess to the world. Healing starts inside, and nobody else can meet you there but God. If nobody else will forgive you, *he* will forgive and accept you. Surrender your shame to him. Sometimes we know we should do things but need confirmation and clarity. God is there for this purpose.

Thirteen

How to Begin, and How It Will Go

Before you begin, it's important to look at your impulses in a new way. Not a negative way, but a way in which you can build a positive relationship with those impulses. You will want to know what to look for and how to deal with it. You will also want to become more aware and learn your tendencies. For men, the tendencies can vary. However, they are generally the same.

It is never "the right time" to start, and your impulse will always keep you from believing it is. Expect the unexpected, and be ready to face the challenge. When dealing with your impulse it is better to expect the worst—and that you will need all the tools to help you succeed. You must over-prepare for the moments you'll come face-to-face with your impulses. Prepare to be alone with the strong feelings of temptation to give in. Always be ready and have a plan. If you learn one way to overcome your impulses, learn another way.

This can get easier. However, it will get harder before it gets easier. Don't fall for the myth that this is an end-all and be-all. The beginning is the hardest. However, once you go a week and then into a month, and more, without sexual release you become stronger and more confident to continue. It does not go away, but once you start to succeed, the once-heavy burden begins to look small. It can get easier, but it is not because you got rid of the impulse. It's because you become better.

To create a positive relationship with your sexual impulse, you must first **start in the mind by changing the story you tell yourself.** Your impulse is no longer something that is feared, but it needs to be understood and respected. Let the impulse in; be aware of it, feel it. This allows you to study what you're up against.

Next is to create a positive relationship: not just mentally but also physically. **Instead of being tense in your body, relax it.** Do not react to your impulse, but sit with it for a moment. Teach your body to accept it through composure. Breathe deep, and be aware of the tension in your body. If there is tension somewhere, breathe deep into that area and relax it. Be present with it and do not react. Rejecting it will backfire. This is a great exercise when you have an impulsive sexual desire. We think this is only sexual energy—until we feel the energy in our body instead of our genitals. Stop what you're doing and embrace it through relaxing your body with deep breathing. Start to disperse the tension from one area of your body and spread it to your entire body by releasing the tense spot and visualizing the energy spreading.

YOUR IMPULSE IS A MASTER MANIPULATOR

If you tolerate impulsive sex in any way, you will fail. You must make the decision to go cold turkey with all forms of sex.

Reject all excuses. Excuses can be the biggest distractions. Most may seem relevant, but they are not. We will make something like giving up sex or a sacrifice much bigger than it has to be. We make it so important we forget we are enslaved and in chains through our impulse. This journey is a journey of change, so you can be rewarded with freedom; however, it is important to embrace the change. The change is mainly a new way of living with your impulse, and rather than trying to kill it, you create a new identity with it. You seek to identity with it in a positive and productive way. You will learn much about your sexual impulse on your journey, but you must keep an open mind because it might not react the way you think it will. Your impulse, however, is not only relentless but also a manipulator. It will turn your excuses into big problems and bigger distractions. Most men fail to overcome their impulse not because they don't know what they are fighting, but because they don't know the depth of what they are fighting.

In the beginning, distractions are just distractions. Just like if you are sailing and your boat is sinking because of weight, you must get rid of all things of low value. You don't have time to justify what to keep or not keep or you will sink. Disregard all silly excuses, or you will act out of impulse through sex every time. Expect the unexpected excuses and expect the illusion of importance caused by your impulse. Get ready for the manipulating mindset that will make something small into something big. As humans we want to make decisions *now*, or at least as soon as possible. Once you understand your impulse can deceive your mind, then you think twice. You must stay grounded and not react. One of the best strategies and tools you can use is to give at least a day before making a decision to make sure you are not reacting to your impulse. Never justify or make a decision out of anxiety. You have to be firm in your mission when it comes to different areas of your life as well, because your impulse is part of you. You can trigger and affect it through outside sources. Be okay with your impulse attempting to manipulate your thoughts. You want to learn to let your impulse flow without acting to it. See it, recognize it, but don't react to it. Try to understand its trickery, and you will be able to read it every time it shows up.

Your impulse will be convincing. When you act out sexually, it has become justified in the mind. You have decided to go through with it. Usually a man trying to recover goes through a series of back-and-forth statements in a type of inner dialogue that, sometimes, he is barely aware of. The man wants to recover, but the impulse is very persuasive. The man's impulse alone cannot get him to act out sexually, or it would already have been done. The man's impulse needs the man's consciousness to agree. The justification is never just a one-sided thing, but the impulse and the conscience have to both make the decision, together, to act out. The conscience may be hesitant, but if you relapse it is because your conscience allowed itself to be led by your impulse.

A common excuse goes something like this: "I should work on my project so I can finish it on time." The impulse may say: "You have been working hard enough; you need a break." You may say, "A break sounds nice." Your impulse may say, "Nobody's around and you can go to your favorite porn site." You may say, "But I need to stop acting out and make it at least a week." Your impulse may say, "Well, it's only been one day." And so on. The feeling of your impulse will drown out your dialogue if you let it. Your impulse will seek to be louder and relentless—but you should be even louder so you can free yourself of it.

START WITH MASSIVE ACTION

Humans are creatures of habit. To change the common habits, you have to disrupt them, and sometimes, in order to change, you need to do things abruptly, with force. To change your impulsive cycle you must make an abrupt change. Shock the system. Disrupt the pattern. It becomes the cry for help that turns into action.

Do not be afraid to "act irrationally" to overcome your impulse. I encourage you to shut out all access to sexual release—forcefully if you can. Seeing yourself make these changes is a great way to begin to break the habit and sends a subconscious message to yourself that you are indeed serious and, because of your action, will inherently desire to want to overcome even more. No mere thought or feeling, no matter how strong, will change you. Action is stronger than words, thoughts, or feelings ever will be.

Forcefully shutting out all access to sexual release for yourself could look like: ending your sexual relationship, whatever kind of relationship that is; destroying your electronic device that you watch pornography with; destroying sexual property including condoms, lubricant, things of that nature; putting a porn blocker on your computer; paying someone to help keep yourself accountable; paying for a program. The list can go on and on. You have likely noticed that I used the words *force* and *destroy*. That is not a mistake. Action reinforces the conviction in your brain, especially action that is perceived as sincere. I call this "massive action." If you value thirty dollars' worth of condoms or a thousand-dollar flat-screen TV more than freedom from yourself, then I challenge you to rethink and prioritize what is important to you.

You must make these changes quickly. If you know what you must do, then do it without hesitation. Use your impulsive power, this time for good. Deciding what you must do can be pretty simple; sticking to the decision can be entirely different. You must act quickly. Your impulse is a deceiver, and one of the best ways to overcome it is to not give it a chance to deceive you. You must make the changes before your impulse makes you change your mind. Make your change as permanent as possible. When you make the change, make it so that you cannot bring things back to the way they were, or least make it very difficult to bring them back to the way they were. As soon as you start asking yourself if you will regret this change, it's already too late. You will not regret this decision, but feel empowered because of it. Make the change and make it fast.

You will also want to make more than one change. Our impulse is likely to think of other avenues in which to find sexual release. Recognize this and be willing to adjust to making another change as well. This is the dirty but truly necessary work that needs to be done. It is ripping off of the Band-Aid when you want to hesitate.

You are fighting a battle. The most important battle. The internal battle: both mental and spiritual. You are destroying or weakening all

THIS BATTLE IS NOT FOR WIMPS, BUT FOR A FIERCE MAN. parts of you that cause your impulse to destroy, and you are also strengthening and lifting up all other parts of you that you use to fight with. This battle is not for wimps, but for a fierce man. If you are not a fierce man now, then fight hard and you will be one. There is always something to fight for. This is your battle. Let it strengthen you and transform you.

Don't face it alone. You are now smarter than that. You should fear being unprepared, so you should be over-prepared. There are many ways to prepare yourself, and one is through changing your environment to "high ground." Face your impulse only on your terms, where you have the advantage. The easier you can access sexual release in any moment, the bigger advantage your impulse has. You will have a bigger craving for sexual release when your environment is suggesting sexual release. Whatever your impulsive tendencies are, you may have a bigger craving if you are around them: a person, store, form of technology, being alone, social media, website, seeing a picture, or even a location where you have an impulsive memory.

When exposed to the triggers, you face a disadvantage. When away from these triggers or even anything that allows you access to the triggers, you have an advantage. It's just like craving food when you're hungry. If you see it in front of you, or see anything that reminds you of food, the greater your craving will be and the harder time you're going to have when trying not to indulge your craving. You will learn to run to a better environment, away from your triggers. For example, if you are triggered by social media and you're around the computer that you watch pornography on, you will want to make sure your environment is away from that computer, and maybe even turn off your phone. Do not surrender to your impulse by giving in to the beginning stages of it. Either escape and re-engage with the advantage, or lose because you gave your impulse the upper hand.

The other suggestion for sexual release is your feelings. Some of your feelings may be a trigger to release your sexual tension, like the feeling of being alone, angry, upset, sad, and other things of that nature. Recognize these and take action to avoid these disadvantages. Now you can fight on your own terms, whether that is through your location or a new, changed emotional state. If you know that your impulse has an advantage when you're alone or angry, you know to either adjust those feelings or recognize them as a trigger and escape to an environment where you, instead, have the advantage. If you feel alone or angry, phone a friend, work out, take a break, meditate, change your state in your body, or hang out somewhere in town. The whole idea is to realize when you are triggered or likely to be triggered and to act quickly so you don't end up giving in to your impulse.

Act quickly and change your attitude and emotional state, if possible, and put yourself in a better environment. Don't keep yourself in an environment full of temptation, and don't make it harder on yourself. Just leave or avoid it. Maybe you are feeling upset and want to indulge in pornography. Instead, decide to go for a walk in town; this helps clear your head and changes your state, making you less upset while also placing yourself in a far better environment. When walking through town it is far less likely that you will end up watching pornography. And therefore, of course, you have put your impulse at a disadvantage. It can no longer affect you the same as when you are alone in a secluded room with access to triggers and easy sexual release. Your impulse will have to get you to head back to your secluded room, and that will be much harder. Not impossible, but it will create a buffer—which is sometimes all you need to get your head straight.

Be aware of your tendencies, learn to feel your impulses, and know when to escape to higher ground. Because of this greater awareness, you will have a greater acceptance of yourself as a man by accepting your true feelings and tendencies of expression without reacting negatively and focusing on them as insecurities. To advance into better consciousness, you should no longer judge your feelings or react, but instead diagnose them. Use your feelings and reactions to indicate whether you should prepare for battle or not. Yes, your impulsive feelings often seem like they come from nowhere; however, most of the time they come from some type of physical or mental trigger. Once you become aware of your triggers, you must become aware of the feelings and thoughts associated with sexual desire. Learn to feel the energy in your body. It is easy to find yourself in the wrong place at the wrong time when you are unaware of these feelings. When you catch them early you have time to make the easier decision by saying no to your impulse, and to start preparing for it by either changing your emotional state or changing your environment—or better yet, doing both. Recognize the rise of your sexual desire and make a decision to change your situation. Your desire is like a monster that never gets full. Every sexual thought or suggestion, direct or indirect, feeds your desire and will be eaten up, only to make it grow bigger and seem much stronger. Never lead on your desire, but recognize it before it becomes stronger and harder to stop.

You must never ignore it. Many men try to continue their task in the moment and work right through it. When they feel their impulse growing, they ignore it and continue what they were doing. This can make the impulse worse. We think this may be a successful way of handling it, but it depends what kind of work you're doing. To battle it you must not engage it, but you also need to not engage anything that triggers the feelings associated with it that cause the stirring of your impulse. Feelings that stir your impulse can often be anger and loneliness, and one larger trigger still can be general stress. Most men have learned to cope with stress through sexual release. In these cases, every time the brain experiences stress, it associates sexual release as a means of escape. One

> YOU MUST NEVER IGNORE IT. MANY MEN TRY TO CONTINUE THEIR TASK IN THE MOMENT AND WORK RIGHT THROUGH IT.

of the biggest changes you can the make next time is to discontinue your activities that cause even the smallest amount of stress, and work instead to calm down your stress and impulse. The strategy of battling your impulse by letting it settle down can be extremely effective.

Your impulse is like a beast. Once it's awake and agitated, it is uncontrollable. It is only controllable when it is calm and asleep. Most men do not know how to properly calm their impulse—or don't think it possible. As I said, it is common for men to try to ignore their impulse and continue engaging in current tasks. Usually even a simple task will cause enough stress to agitate your impulse to the point where you lose control and relapse. (Some men go back to their tasks too early.)

To take a step back from your task, change your environment and state of emotion, and then going back to your stressful task can make the difference between feeling in control or not. There are times you may return without feeling the impulse at all. This is a great practice: for men to take a step back from their triggers, and life as well, to see and think more clearly. This will rejuvenate a man's perspective, refresh his state of emotion, clear his head, and calm his impulse. It is normal for men to be task-oriented, always focused on a project and being as productive and efficient as possible. Men don't want to stop working on their project because it's easy to feel as if they are wasting time if they do so. It is only when we actually step back and disengage in our task-oriented mindset that we realize how unproductive we actually are by "trying" to be productive. The task-oriented mindset makes a man spread himself too thin, and most men end up indulging in more sexual release than they would have because of the amount of extra stress, sometimes being the result of hours and hours of wasted time and sexual energy that could have been used productively. You have probably noticed that when your impulse is alive and growing, if you try to stay focused on your task your stress seems to multiply, causing your reaction to engage in your impulse to become more intense.

*"Tasks don't get a man anywhere more conscious or free
than he is capable of being in this present moment."*
–DAVID DEIDA, *THE WAY OF THE SUPERIOR MAN*

During this journey you will find de-stressing activities that work for you. These activities either don't cause you the stress that will normally trigger you or they do not feed your impulse. You can measure how triggered your impulse is by feeling the increase or decrease of its intense feeling.

A way of looking at disengaging your impulse is like how most people deal with a fever. When you have a fever you do not usually work or strain yourself but instead "fever it out." You wait for your body and the fever to do its thing and calm down. Once you feel better you continue with your activities. Again, ways of disengaging your impulse include taking a walk, meditating, even napping and relaxing. These can be of benefit to you because they help you carve out time to rejuvenate yourself with a refreshing activity, and they remind you to relax and be in the moment. Do something that doesn't strain you mentality. Physical activity is usually okay, but your impulse will likely react more to mental strain. Enjoy a mentally relaxing activity.

When you begin to hit your threshold and are starting to break the habit of your impulse, your body and mind are not used to it. You may feel like you are withdrawing from drugs. Some men feel this experience of withdrawal more, some less, than others. Your impulse has likely become a true addiction. You may begin to feel these withdrawals when you have been a week or a month without sexual release, and you're very near the mark that would break your streak of not acting out. Some will feel

YOU MUST BE READY TO BE YOUR STRONGEST AND SACRIFICE THE MOST AT THE BEGINNING. YOU WILL HAVE TO SACRIFICE YOUR MOOD AS WELL AS, PERHAPS, ONE OR MORE NIGHTS OF SLEEP.

these withdrawals sooner or later. This is the most important part of the journey, and usually the hardest. This is the big climb. Break through this barrier, and hope is waiting for you on the other side. You must be ready to be your strongest and sacrifice the most at the beginning. You will have to sacrifice your mood as well as, perhaps, one or more nights of sleep.

You must be relaxed as you break through this barrier. Like someone who is sick, you will have to wait it out. Especially when attempting to disengage your impulse by relaxing and refreshing yourself. You will find that in the beginning it may take several hours or days of spending your time in mentally refreshing activities before your impulse calms down.

The nice thing is that once you get past the first breakthrough things usually become better, and you will see yourself spending less time having to partake in these mentally effortless activities and "fevering through it." Also, most men can live life normally when going through this personal breakthrough and through feeling the withdrawals and strong temptations to relapse. They usually don't have trouble when they are working their regular job or doing regular chores. There may be stress at work, and your impulse may be building; however, usually work requires you to be attentive, or you are in an environment with people which makes it difficult to relapse. Most of the time you don't need to find "the right environment" because you are already in it at your day job. Now, sometimes men work from home, and if they have found working from home a problem in giving into their impulse, then it is a good idea to either go into work, rent some kind of office, or figure out something else that will make it much more difficult to relapse. The change of your environment can be extremely important and effective. Even if you can still make it happen and find a way to get your sexual release, the fact that it is much harder makes it much easier to say no to your impulse. You probably don't need to take off work to overcome your impulse in the beginning, but if you have to, there is no shame in making that decision.

HAVE A TOOL, A WEAPON; THEN HAVE A PLAN AND STRATEGY

You must be prepared for the next time your impulse comes to life. Your impulse will always come back to life, usually when you are not expecting it. There are many different tools and plans that may be more or less effective for you. Some tools and plans you may discover on your own or through others. It is up to you to apply them and see if they can help you. Never be close-minded about a certain tool or plan. You make dislike one, but just like overcoming your impulse, you have to sacrifice. You have to be willing to give up something as well as disregard your feelings in order to reap the massive benefits of freedom from your impulse.

Humans are creatures who focus. Our mind can wander and seem to redirect itself. Sometimes we try to stop it from wandering, but the wandering only gets worse and more out of control than before. Just like breathwork and meditation, one of the best ways to combat your wandering thoughts is to let them flow—and focus on something else. One way of meditating is by focusing on your breathing to get your mind away from aimless thoughts. When you are face to face with your impulse you usually react by trying to stop the energy and the thoughts it provokes. This is a strategy that you may have already used. What you will find is that this doesn't work very well. It will tend to stimulate a reaction of stress and lack of control. You will lose clarity and your better sense of judgment. Focusing on something else—either a mindset that works or something tangible like an activity—is effective. You aren't trying to shut your brain off; you are changing its focus. Next time you feel your impulse growing, don't shut it out, but feel it and recognize it. Then draw your attention to something specific like the tool or the plan

YOU ARE NOT THE ONE WHO MAKES IT RAIN TO FILL UP THE RIVER, BUT YOU ARE THE ONE WHO CAN DIRECT THE RIVER'S FLOW.

and start feeding this new focus and drawing your attention toward your strategy, which, in effect, will take your focus off your impulsive thoughts and feelings. Learn to let things flow like a river. You are not the one who makes it rain to fill up the river, but you are the one who can direct the river's flow.

To feel the impulse come alive and grow will naturally excite you. It enlivens you with energy and power. It is easy to want to increase that feeling and caress the power of its tension. Most often men do engage it and want to feel the thrill of the arousal. Men, though, engage it in a way of sexual stimulus. Your impulsive feelings become your focus, and you can either let that feed sexual stimulus or some other focus. Don't attempt to stop it, but first feel it throughout your body. It has great potential for creativity and action. Do not react to it yet, but let it touch and inspire every cell of your body. Feel the aliveness—but now direct that feeling elsewhere. You may have been triggered by someone attractive walking by you, or a photo, a thought, or a smell. Whatever it was, don't engage in the sexualized thoughts it provokes, but plan to redirect that focus to be either thinking of or doing something different, meaningful. This is your plan when you are triggered. You may have some plans of focus and action for different triggers, but to succeed you need to know what to do when you're in that unexpected situation.

There are a few ways to redirect your focus. One is adding a quick mental thought that could deter you from sexualizing your focus. When you're triggered and notice sexualizing thoughts, have a plan of go-to thoughts. Take the creativity of the impulsive thoughts and redirect it into nonsexual thoughts. Thoughts of creating or giving. Sexualized thoughts usually revolve around the idea of taking and using. When you start thinking of how to give to that attractive person, your mind becomes free to act differently. Maybe you're triggered by seeing a magazine photo of an immodest image. What to do? Turn it over so it isn't being displayed toward you or other people.

You can use these opportunities to help and inspire other men too. One commonly used plan is to instantly pray for the person you are sexualizing in your mind, praying as soon as you are triggered. Make your intention giving rather than satisfying an unsatisfied desire. Pray; even a short prayer takes focus. It's hard to pray for somebody and want to have sex with them at the same time.

Figure out your go-to activity. The mind can elicit action and, in the same way, action can elicit the mind. Use action that doesn't trigger your impulse nor the emotional triggers to your impulse; for example: anger, loneliness, and stress. Again, action reinforces your beliefs as well as redirects your thoughts. Some kind of action is necessary; even action to decide to relax. The most important part of this plan of action is not to stop your impulse but to stop engaging in its triggers and to start moving away from them. Take your focus off your impulse by focusing on something else. You can decide to work on a task; however, make sure it does not stress you out. Even the smallest bit of stress can easily cause your impulse to abruptly infiltrate your energy and thoughts. Be prepared to drop your task when your impulse arises. You can always go back to it later. It's time to take a break, at least from your stressful tasks. If you don't you will risk the added weight your impulse will have.

Maybe your planned activity is working out, taking a walk, napping, calling a friend, or some other activity. Once you occupy yourself in some other way that works, you will be able to much more easily calm your impulse. The more you do this, the better you get at it. There is no rule on having to engage in the same activities; only as they work and calm your impulse. And switching things up from time to time may be helpful in long-term recovery. Your activity can and should also be your "higher ground," the environment that doesn't contain triggers or access to your impulse and sexual release. During your planned activity you will notice the intensity of your impulse. It doesn't eliminate the way sexual release depletes you, but it settles and calms down. You can still feel the energy of the impulse. It is different from when it was aroused, but it is still there. It fills your body with energy and alertness. It is always ready. Ready to become aroused once more. Calm but alert. There is a certain kind of intensity men get used to. It is not intensity like before, but the lingering power that makes your body feel vibrant and alive but still calm. It is always ready. Most men have never experienced this feeling. Most men are, usually, depleted. Many to most men are never fully alive.

A great deal of the time we know what to do and just don't do it. Even when you have a plan you may know exactly how you should act when triggered, whether that is taking a long walk and praying for your trigger, or something else, but often we don't do it. We should be like the athlete who knows the game is coming or that he will have to take the winning shot when he doesn't expect it, so he trains for it. He goes through the motions like he is in that exact scenario so he is prepared—and so should we. Even when you aren't feeling the impulse spontaneously, practice a few times a day. Pray and go through your plan like you are feeling the intensity and manipulation of your impulse. Practice and train yourself to be ready. Rewire your brain through action. Much of the time men are ashamed when they relapse, and they want to overcome it, but they think they have to wait until they feel it again. Your next opportunity to overcome your impulse doesn't start when your impulse is aroused, but before it is. How you practice is how you perform. Set the stage for your next trial now, never *during* it. Just like a good athlete, you will never be good on your own unless you train and practice.

You control your environment; your environment controls you. How easy is access to your impulsive triggers, and where do you find sexual release? What in your daily life drives you to give in to your impulses and deplete yourself of energy and power? It could be a person, a goal, a problem, or even physical material. Maybe something in your life causes stress, and you have been inclined, in the past, to deplete yourself because of this stress. Maybe it is necessary stress, like your job or daily chores; and maybe it is not. If not, you can consider getting rid of or destroying it, but if it is, you must reduce it and learn to handle the stress. The intensity of your sexual urges can so often be the gauge of the balance in your life. The strength of the intensity is not the problem but the effect of the problem. We think that we need to fix our sexual urge, but instead we need to take another step back and examine what causes the uncontrollable sexual intensity. This can be another tool to find balance in your life. Maybe you're not expending enough energy in your workouts or life purpose; maybe your stress is out of control; maybe something has been making you angry. The truth is we should never use our life circumstances as an excuse. We are always going to be stressed, angry, or have some other undesirable emotion. We will never be balanced, but we can get as close as we can to being balanced, and this can help a man with his sexual urges. Your sexual intensity won't go away, but you can gain a handle on it when you control what your sexual urges react to. You are thinking foolishly when you believe that you have enough strength, by pure willpower on your own, to say no to your impulse while in the heat of its moment. One of the best ways to recover from your impulse is to act as though you are taking care of yourself just as you would somebody else. You will think less of controlling your weak willpower and more about controlling the external effects of your impulse. Yes, you can ask other people to help; however, you must learn to help yourself by creating the boundaries now, *before* you're in the heat of the moment.

Examine your environment and the things you're exposed to on a daily basis. How do you access your habit of sexual release? Is it a person, technology, or place? In the beginning of your journey of recovering you will need to open your eyes. You will need to become aware of the details of your impulsive habits. Follow the path to getting to your habits, and find ways to put obstacles in the way of your impulse. You are the father to yourself; child-proof your journey for abundant success. Do not interfere and scold yourself, but lovingly guide yourself on this journey toward the light and toward becoming a man. When you don't have the father you need, you become him. Pornography is the most easily accessible path of finding stimulation. The biggest problem with pornography is its accessibility. How can you prevent the accessibility? Putting obstacles in your way is something you don't do lightly. You place the obstacles abruptly and radically. Learn the ways of your impulse and remind yourself of the deceiver and trickster that it is. Don't give your impulsive side a chance to breathe.

Get rid of your relationships and all the people you have on the back burner for hookups. Delete their phone numbers, all contact info, all social media. Delete all the nudes you have on your phone, the addresses, messages, etc. Destroy or alter the material or device which leads you to your impulse. Put a blocker for all pornography on your computer and phone. Switch your phone to a flip phone; be creative! At first it doesn't matter whether you can still access sexual release or not. The entire point is to make accessing it as difficult as possible. Don't be afraid to go overboard. The minute you show mercy to the part of your impulsive mentality you are trying to change is the minute you fall for its trap. If you're still finding a way to access sexual release through your relationships and devices after this, then keep going and continue to put obstacles in your way, going until you find those that work. You will have to make sacrifices. Figure out what those sacrifices are. Make those sacrifices so you can have a better future.

After you get rid of your access to sexual release, it's time to analyze what triggers get you to the point of this release. You are like a detective who needs to find a pattern. What triggers your sexual urges? It could be anything, and often even something, unrelated to sex. Of course you have your emotional triggers; however, it could be a nonsexual thought, sound, music, smell, memory, or other thing. Maybe it's a particular time during the day when you get home from work or are alone at home. Most often, though, we are triggered by something related to sex like a picture in a magazine or one on social media. First, find your trigger, then add obstacles between you and it; if you are triggered when you get home from work, change the pattern. Don't go straight home after work, or, have a definite plan when you get there. If you are triggered from being home alone, go to an office and get things done. If you are triggered by pictures or social media, get rid of the pictures. I would highly recommend either limiting your access to social media or getting rid of it altogether. Unfollow the people who post pictures that trigger you. The fact is you may not be able to get rid of all the sexually stimulating triggers in your life; however, you can control your exposure to them and create new habits to avoid them. Maybe you look forward to spending your time looking at someone's pictures on social media or being home alone, but again, you will have to make sacrifices if you want to get better. You don't choose if you want to better yourself after your recovery; you have to better yourself to recover. Many of our triggers have become their own addictions. Avoid these triggers; limit them as much as possible.

You need to make changes and adjustments for the new man that is in the making. Your impulsive behavior is the child that needs to grow up. Throw away the porn pacifier. Make your home and life trigger-proof. You get what you negotiate in life and what you negotiate with your impulse. If you allow impulsive access to sexual release, it will take full advantage. Create boundaries and make access to your sexual stimulus impossible. Get rid of TV shows and the pictures that trigger you. Go to bed early so you don't find yourself in the exact situation you have been trying to prevent.

> THROW AWAY THE PORN PACIFIER. MAKE YOUR HOME AND LIFE TRIGGER-PROOF. YOU GET WHAT YOU NEGOTIATE IN LIFE.

Always be on your guard. Most of the time you will find yourself getting rid of bad habits. Don't just get rid of the bad habits, replace them with good ones. Use this journey as an opportunity for personal change. You need to disrupt your old identity by creating a new one.

A bottom line: sacrifice safety and comfort. Men are trapped in protecting themselves from the outside world and their true reality as a man. They hide in their secret habits, covering up reality and numbing themselves to life. Men who indulge their impulses risk their potential and greatness. Their impulse is their coping method, their adult pacifier, their secret way of dealing with the reality of their truth and the wounds of life, never giving themselves a chance to overcome them. These men suffer in silence and don't grow because they face no actual challenges. Their unsatisfied life allows them to get lost in ever more comfort and indulgence. It becomes a habit and cycle. To disrupt your cycle you need some type of impact, something to break the cycle.

Fourteen

Tools and Techniques

There are many tools and tricks that can help a man along this journey. Some are more helpful than others, but it is up to the man to use them so they can assist his will in overcoming his impulse. A tool can make a big difference, but it is not the cure or the final piece to the puzzle. A tool is only a support mechanism to the main decision. It is there to make a man stronger and more effective than before. The use and practice of these tools is putting the decision into practice.

Thinking *I just have to do this or that to quit* is not the right mentality. All techniques and practices are there to reinforce new beliefs, thought patterns, and stories that lead to a true conviction to change our habits. Understand it isn't one technique that fixes your problem. However, one or more may be the focus for the intention you need to help convict you to change. Just like working out, this is a muscle, and you need to strengthen it or it will get weaker. I have witnessed men who haven't relapsed to sex for years still practicing the tools and techniques that got them to recovery. These men make the tools and habits and use them as though their recovery journey started yesterday. If this isn't your top priority, it won't work. The first breakthrough will take the most work. It may take a little less work with time, but still, always ride the wave and stay consistent.

The discipline to consistently use your tools and techniques is very important. Again, action reinforces your beliefs and the decisions you made in the beginning. It is not so much how effective these tools are but that, when you practice them, they remind you of your faithfulness and determination toward your commitment. Besides the advantage and edge, these tools lead you to the continual practices to actively pursue and apply these techniques that deepen your conviction toward your decision. Without the sincere decision that every tool and technique is based on, all is useless. *Both decision and sacrifice are the backbone of recovery.* You have all the power within you to say no to your impulse. You need to convince yourself that you want this, and it starts with action and sacrifice in applying yourself to the techniques.

Through the main portion of this chapter, I'm going to outline some great tools and strategies to help you overcome. Look for the key statements in **bold type**.

First and foremost, you must share your impulsive behavior, express it, by telling someone about it. What this does is allow shame to be exposed to light. Do not be afraid to show the world. Shame tends to hide. It does not seek healing, but self-loathing. It is normal to feel shame from sexually impulsive slavery because you know something is inherently wrong, and it can be embarrassing to share it. As we know, this feeling can cause a cycle, and a common way to cope with the down periods in this cycle is self-indulgence, and this does nothing but usually result in habitual sexual release. Shame does not serve you but repeats the cycle and affirms your habitual identity. Talk about it with your male friends, therapists, and groups.

I would not recommend you share this with your girlfriend or wife. Even though you are on a good path toward personal transformation, it is not worth causing her to resent you. You don't need to tell the woman in your life everything. If she makes it seem as though you should tell her everything, she is revealing needy and insecure behavior. It's time to grow up and for both of you to be capable independents for the sake of the relationship. And it starts with you. You can tell women about your impulsive behavior. However, be aware that some women may never understand it like men will.

When sharing with supportive listeners, you must be okay with looking in the dark places of your impulse, the places where it hurts. Revealing these will help you heal and start to construct a plan to get out of your situation.

Find people who will listen to you about your impulsive behavior and support your recovery. If you can't find anybody or need more support, join a Sexaholics Anonymous group. There are groups all around the country, and nowadays you can Zoom to join from anywhere. Their program works if you do it sincerely. The support and affirmation from others fuels your conviction.

> SEE YOUR IMPULSIVENESS AS IT IS, NOT MORE OR LESS THAN IT IS. YOU HAVE TO KNOW THE REALITY OF YOUR PROBLEM.

Typically men will inflate or deflate the reality of their situation, only to realize this after sharing it. It was either bigger or smaller than they thought it was. See your impulsiveness as it is, not more or less than it is. You have to know the reality of your problem. You can't effectively aim for a goal without knowing and accepting your current position relative to that goal. Accept where you are and move forward from there. You can write about it and express it that way; however, this is not as healing as sharing it with others. It takes courage and humility to share it with others, and it becomes profoundly beneficial to your recovery.

Also extremely important: **do not shame or punish yourself.** Practice the habit of not punishing or feeling guilty for yourself, especially after you have given in to your impulse. One of the best ways to train to overcome your impulse is to prevent yourself from continuing to indulge after the first sexual release. Men shame themselves, and this only works to get them to attempt to cover up their shame in the next numbing sexual experience. Forgive yourself after your lack of success, and keep on forgiving yourself with, of course, the intention of change.

When you slip and fall, get up immediately. The real opportunity for growth presents itself after your first ejaculation. This is an opportunity for maturity. You either teach yourself the consistency that will give you success, or you teach yourself the inconsistent mindset of muscling through it and then indulging like crazy. That mindset may seem to work; however, it will not last long. Learn how to live with your sexual energy by never being fully depleted. The streak seems nice, but when you trip up, indulging in your impulse will only make your attachment and desire for release even greater. It's not so much about whether you will be knocked down or not, but about how long you stay down. Men easily get hooked on how long they can go without sexual release, but when they slip up and relapse, they don't think it counts anymore, so they make the mistake of then binging.

> IT'S NOT SO MUCH ABOUT WHETHER YOU WILL BE KNOCKED DOWN OR NOT, BUT ABOUT HOW LONG YOU STAY DOWN.

Just as with a diet, even if you cheat once on it, you have to return to the goal you started with. Your binging reinforces that this food means a lot to you and makes you more likely to binge in the future. Recovering from your impulse is like riding a bull. After you fall off the bull, you need to get back on it. You cannot just stay on the ground or you'll get stomped on; you will relapse again. To get back on the bull will take effort. Sprint away from your triggers, take a walk, call a friend—any of the things we discussed in the previous chapter. You must change your state of mind by changing and influencing it with new activities. Do not indulge yourself in other forms of craving like binge eating or binging on social media. Doing this leaves you in a weak state of mind, making you more likely not to withstand the next temptation that comes your way, and causing you to relapse once more.

Tell yourself a new story. Your impulse over-promises, deceives, and over-exaggerates your sexual experience. To be tricked by your impulse is like being a child in a fantasy world. It isn't real, and what you imagine isn't as hyped up as it seems, and it is leaving out the shame and regret that will come. It's a child's fantasy that is just in your imagination. You imagine it bringing you satisfaction and relief from your current stress, loneliness, or other negative emotion. It will not satisfy you but leave you unsatisfied and looking for more. Adults still believe in and are tricked by this fantasy, many of them almost every time. The problem is that instead of reminding ourselves of the truth about this fantasy, we indulge in it; it sounds so good that we are sold by it. Someone responsible may have the same tendencies as a child, but he is mature enough to realize the lie behind them. Remind yourself of the truth and the fake satisfaction that you get from your impulse.

Tell yourself the positive story of overcoming your impulse and re-inforcing recovery by reminding yourself of the truth of that impulse, how it will leave you in a worse situation than before. It's time to reveal the truth about your fantasy. It's not easy, but you need to see it and be reminded for the betterment of your maturity.

An effective new story is convincing. Think, journal, and talk about it. Imagine that you are in a courtroom pleading your case by using logical, thorough arguments that make sense to you. Dig deeper for better understanding of yourself and how you can make better sense of your situation. Work to create no doubt in your mind and then connect this story to your creed of who you are as a person. Make sure there is no argument that will convince you otherwise. You must have a counter for all objections you might give in to so you can understand yourself. The objections could be seeking sex to reaffirm self-worth, find love, or cope with stress.

Prevent yourself from being impaired, and be on your guard at all times. One helpful tactic is to create momentum and continue to feed off your success. It is super important to be ready to alter your impulse—whether you had the most stressful day at work or it is 2 a.m. and you are unable to think straight. We can find ourselves in situations where we naturally feel impaired because of our mood or health. Alcohol and drugs are conscious choices to make oneself impaired. One night of drinking or smoking can make you relapse and disrupt your momentum. Learn to control your impulse without being impaired first. You must be able to handle your impulse even under natural stress before trying to allow drinking back into your life—but definitely not *while* you are still struggling with it. Getting rid of drinking, drugs, and even other activities may be another huge sacrifice you need to make. And maybe you need to sacrifice something forever. A sacrifice is just another value of yours that you need to trade in for the prize you really want.

One general rule, even for life, is to find out what you can and can't do. What does and doesn't bring you over the edge. These could be hobbies, activities, friends, or other things that are unnecessary for your life and cause you pain, loss of control, excessive anxiousness, anger, and more. You are unique, and this is okay. It's just like a person allergic to peanuts; he doesn't come anywhere near eating peanuts. He doesn't take it personally, because he understands other people have unique situations like his. It doesn't mean he can't eat other foods. In the same way, it doesn't mean there aren't other friends, activities, and hobbies out there for you.

Watch your anxiety. Your anxiety can be a gauge of your sexual energy. It can also be a huge trigger. Control your anxiety and be in tune with it. A big part of recovery is awareness. It is extremely important to be consistent with clear-cut steps that help you recover as well

CONTROL YOUR ANXIETY AND BE IN TUNE WITH IT. A BIG PART OF RECOVERY IS AWARENESS.

as reading signs and cues that tell you to take precautions to prevent relapse. The truth is that there will always be an opportunity to relapse during recovery and beyond, even when you made all access to relapse difficult. You have to know when to reclaim all focus and run away, if necessary. Sometimes you may *physically* have to run from your impulse to prevent a likely relapsing situation. To do that, you need to know how to catch your impulse early and when to run away. This will take time and practice; however, this can be pretty simple and done by changing your focus and measuring your sexual energy as well as your current emotional state. Recognize that you have anxiety at the moment, and when you get triggered by anxiety, it will be your cue to action. Action must be taken immediately. Measure your emotions and figure out what triggers you, whether that is anxiety, anger, loneliness, or some other emotion. Anxiety seems to be an extremely common trigger these days. Are you getting aroused easily, or are you feeling the anticipation of arousal?

Get your emotions in order as much as possible. No, they won't be perfect, but this will help. As soon as you feel anxiety, recognize it and do things that help. You have control over your emotions. Yes, you will feel anxious sometimes; however, you can reduce this, and there are healthy methods of dealing with anxiety like diet, exercise, sleep, friends, and more. Create balance in your life. *Fill your basic physical, mental, and spiritual needs.*

Replace the habits you want to change. Positive change is not so much about getting rid of, but replacing, the bad with the good. One of the best ways to get rid of a thought is not to ignore it but to focus on an alternative thought. Men enslaved to their sexual impulses are also enslaved to the time the sexual impulse takes from them. You are not just getting rid of your impulse but replacing it. And you are also not getting rid of its power and energy but using it elsewhere. Your impulse hasn't been paying its rent. It's time to replace the time and energy that your impulse uses with something other than sexual thoughts or activities. You may find yourself walking more, biking more, and filling your time with activities you have been wanting to do for a while.

Be creative. Men so often expand on their art when aroused, through creating, whether that is painting, writing, music, or just being an artist in their own way. An impulsive mind craves expression, not in the boring, empty tasks but in something that is inspiring in the moment. The way men lose themselves in giving in to their impulse can be turned to losing themselves in art. No matter if you are the worst artist in the world; your mind can create. So drop your chores and explore something creative. You can always go back to the chores later. If you relapse, you will be forced to take a break from your chores and tasks anyway.

Create a habit of prayer. Besides the spiritual benefits, you are basically rehearsing your desire to succeed to yourself, convicting yourself even more. Prayer strengthens your ability to focus even when there are distracting thoughts. It creates a mindset of proactive acceptance and surrender that will assist in helping you persevere without punishing yourself. Pray at least in the morning, afternoon, and night, refocusing yourself on the mission. Memorize prayers, and continue to ask for forgiveness and strength.

Get through to your impulsive side earlier. Our impulse seems to take over our bodies and minds, something like being possessed. We are laser-focused on feeding our impulses and finding sexual release. It feels almost unstoppable, extremely hard for us to get through. When you are "conscious" and truly desire to recover, you want to know how to get through to your impulsive side when it is seemingly in possession of you and out of control. It's like you're sending messages to, and trying to convince your future self not to, indulge in your impulse, that this it is a bad and dangerous idea. You may just want to scream at yourself and tell your impulse no, but it is not that easy. You must instead set the stage for yourself, maybe leaving a note on your computer or mirror that is a quote or saying that reminds you to focus. You can also block your access, as we have said, through a porn blocker; there are many types and strategies here. Men relapse not so much because they didn't have control but because they weren't fully present and focused on their desire to overcome their impulse.

Rewards are a great way to influence yourself to recover. As humans we look forward to and are motivated by rewards. Sometimes just the beginning stages of freedom from our impulses are not enough to encourage us to proceed. You may catch yourself negotiating whether it is worth continuing to recover or not. You may debate whether the pleasure and irresponsibility will feel better than the freedom and power you will gain from recovering. Making a reward for yourself acts as another way to reinforce your commitment. It is a great technique to use because it is an easy, tangible reward. When you have never truly experienced the impactful rewards of being free from your impulse for months, and even years, it is difficult to imagine and anticipate the inherent rewards. It's hard to fight for something if you don't know exactly what you're fighting for and what it feels like. When you create a tangible reward, the goal seems so much more appealing.

> YOU MAY DEBATE WHETHER THE PLEASURE AND IRRESPONSIBILITY WILL FEEL BETTER THAN THE FREEDOM AND POWER YOU WILL GAIN FROM RECOVERING.

One other technique that will help you is to become better at relaxing in your impulse and not just rejecting it. It's best to choose a simple reward. Something that doesn't take lots of preparation and that you won't indulge in before you have earned the reward. Maybe you can't find a good one, and that is still okay. Take the opportunity to put aside time to acknowledge your achievement. Your reward could be as simple as enjoying a bike ride, taking a warm bath, or watching some movies you haven't had time for. Your reward could also be something on a different scale, like going out to your favorite restaurant, throwing a party, or giving yourself an allowance to spend on your hobby.

Get as creative as you want. However, it is still important to keep some type of balance. Celebrate hard, but don't use this as an excuse to over-indulge elsewhere. You can have a reward for every time you make it a week without giving in to your impulse, and maybe a bigger one when you make it to a month or year. It's easy to degrade our achievements. Don't be afraid to realize both the great importance of your recovery and the taking back of your life, as well as making sure you express your gratitude through rewarding yourself.

Empty your bladder. You may have already experienced the effectiveness of urinating when you have a sexual urge. It doesn't make it go away, but it can decrease how stimulated you are quickly and effectively. Pressure around the genital area can cause stimulation to trigger more arousal. To urinate immediately when you are aroused can be extremely beneficial because it makes a difference right away. It takes awareness to know when you are aroused and if emptying your bladder will be helpful. This is one of the first things you can practice when you notice strong feelings of arousal. Get in the habit of acting quickly. After urination, this does not mean you should go right back to what you were doing before. Continue to act on your impulse with the other tools and techniques.

Move, jump for joy, and beat your chest. This can be a super effective way to combat your impulse when triggered. Once you feel the sexual energy surging through your body, you react to it physically instead of sexually. Express it physically like you would express it sexually—with spontaneous force and engagement. Do sprints, dance like a maniac, beat your chest like a barbarian. Act out physically and aggressively. This is redirecting your sexual energy (which we will talk more about in the next chapter). Do this, and the power of your sexual impulse will calm and settle. The more you practice this redirection, the better you will get.

Avoid your triggers. Avoid triggers personal to you as well as the obvious ones like revealing pictures or even music that talks of sexual experiences. Be aware of the common triggers you encounter during your day; learn to avoid them as much as possible. Whatever you are exposing yourself to, you will identify more with. When your attention is directed in some way, you enjoy the energy manifest in wanting and hoping more for it. Everything we experience has an influence on us that may not affect us in the moment, but it definitely will down the line.

Stopping feeding your triggers. It is inevitable that you will encounter triggers. You will run into them or think of them; however, the more you engage your triggers, the more you will want to keep engaging them. When you feed your triggers, they get hungrier and hungrier. Usually, the first thought for men is not to ejaculate but to *engage in one of the triggers,* especially if it is a thought or something physical. Obviously, you want to stay clear of engaging in your triggers, but at first you may catch yourself knee-deep in them. By that point, you are very stimulated, and the desire for your impulse is probably very strong, to the point you feel sick by it. *Time without your triggers will do the trick.* You need to buy yourself time. The intense desire caused by the trigger may not go away instantly, but give it time and it will. Be willing to trade a day and even more to recover. The strong tension may last, but it's up to you to wait it out. The impulse will clear you of clarity and make you mentally sick, but this sickness won't last even when it seems like it will.

When you have a strong urge, it feels like it will not go away. Don't fall for the illusion your impulse plays on you, that it won't go away. The more you feed into it with thoughts or images, the longer it will last.

And conversely, the more you work on these techniques by finding an activity in a safe place with low mental stress, you can multiply that by time, and it will go away.

Escape to high ground. Avoid being vulnerable around your impulse. Sometimes the simplest and most effective technique is to run away from your vulnerable place, whether that is at home or somewhere else alone somewhere. Run like you've never run before. Run like a wild man who won't give in. The sacrifice is to drop everything you're doing, all the chores and tasks, and handle your impulse by escaping to higher ground. This may be hard to do because you feel like you're wasting time, but when you engage in your impulse and fail to drop your tasks to save yourself, you will end up wasting the same amount of time—sometimes even more—by leaving all your tasks for later and engaging in your impulse instead. Drive somewhere; go out into the rain or snow. Anywhere is better than a place where you are vulnerable with your impulse. Your impulse will affect you, but it's up to you to decide how it's going to affect you. Are you willing to negotiate sexual slavery for wasted time and gas so you will not feel bad about yourself?

> THE SACRIFICE IS TO DROP EVERYTHING YOU'RE DOING, ALL THE CHORES AND TASKS, AND HANDLE YOUR IMPULSE BY ESCAPING TO HIGHER GROUND.

Stay busy. You've probably heard it said that "idle hands are the devil's workshop." This, again, is about maintaining as much balance in your life as you can. Do not overwork, but do not underwork. Staying busy can make things easier. Too much free time can make way for too many opportunities to relapse. Being busy may make you feel like you can rest from your impulse, especially when it feels like it won't go away.

When you are triggered, feed your mind with self-talk. Repeat positive and encouraging messages to yourself to overcome your impulses. It's like you are trying to get through to your unreceptive subconscious and can only get through with repetition and sincerity. The impulse seems to take over your thoughts, so you must keep encouraging and motivating yourself to where you actually want to be. Be louder in your head than in your impulse. Drown out the impulse with motivating self-talk. Feed your conscious mind so it will overcome the trigger.

In the end, it is super simple. Continue to feed your desire to recover, practice the steps and techniques so you can calm your impulse, and wait it out.

Increase your sense of self-worth. Do not judge yourself but create habits that support you. Do the things you love. Take care of your body and mind. Exercise, eat healthy, and expose yourself to things that encourage and inspire you. Hang around people who love you.

Continue to learn and grow. Your impulse is always waiting for a chance to be let loose—uncontrollably if possible. It is never over, and you will need new and fresh tools and techniques to keep your impulse at bay.

In the end, to succeed you have to do what works and stop looking for the magic pill that doesn't exist. This book is not going to cure you, but it can help you make the application of the decisions, sacrifices, and consistent actions needed to recover. Do what other people who've had success are doing. You are not different. Yes, you may find tricks that help you more than others; however, it is the daily practice of tools, techniques, and plans that really make you succeed. *One technique is not the solution; instead, use all of the techniques—are all part of the solution.* Just as when you are building a skill, it is going to take time and effort. Most of recovering is doing the actions, every day, that you can and continuing to learn and feed your mind with the knowledge and support needed to persevere. Your mind and conviction will follow your actions.

Don't give up. It is super easy to get discouraged. Maybe it's been years that you've been struggling with this. Or you have tried all the tools and techniques and it hasn't worked out. Many men have taken years to recover, sometimes being sex-free for a year and then falling back into the habits they were in before. Remember, *this is a transformation.* Trying to tweak or fix your impulse is not sustainable. When you fully take responsibility in one area of your life, it is connected to other parts of your life as well. Recognize that transformation often needs to take time. Whenever you go without your impulse for a few days or weeks, and then relapse, it is not for nothing. It is you reinforcing the new, transformed version of yourself. Never lose faith if you feel stuck. Keep expanding yourself in every way possible. Support the best part of you and work on any area that might negatively influence your impulse in an indirect way. Work on your life, relationships, and health. The alternative to a positive attitude toward your impulse will very likely make it worse. Keep using the tools and techniques and reinforcing your decision by surrounding yourself with like-minded people and expanding yourself through learning.

It is exhausting to fight a battle that you keep losing. It destroys your joy and worsens your mood. It would feel better to win at least a little. Men come up with conclusions in their head like they will stop trying or will focus on something else, but that is because they are sick of being sick. They want to run away from their reality of failing—but that will not help them. You can ignore the problem, but it is still there and will come back to bite you. Do not ignore the truth that you genuinely don't want to give up porn or sex, because if you ignore the truth you will never overcome it. You must be okay with your failures and who you are. Do not try to change truth. Do not come up with a new conclusion. Do not give up. Hold on. This is when to be kind to yourself. Help yourself to be in the right state of mind by means other than sexual release.

DATING AND SEX

IF YOU GIVE YOUR IMPULSE AN INCH, IT WILL TAKE A MILE; THAT IS JUST THE POWER AND THE NATURE BEHIND IT. IT IS A MANIPULATOR.

Everybody will be in a different position when they begin their recovery journey, whether they are married, dating, or single. The questions that come up are: should I still have sex with my wife, and should I keep dating even if it is an abstinent relationship? Once you truly understand the nature of your impulse, it will be clear what to do. If you give your impulse an inch, it will take a mile; that is just the power and the nature behind it. It is a manipulator. It is nothing you can negotiate with. You may have tried, in the past, to negotiate with your impulse, but it will get you to cross the line that you set for yourself and were never supposed to cross. The way to heal is to go cold turkey. To avoid sex at all costs. You may put the beast—your impulse—to sleep; however, the only really effective way to reverse its control over yourself is to starve it.

In marriage, your wife doesn't need sex to have a healthy attraction and relationship with you. She needs intimacy, not an orgasm. You and your wife can build that intimacy by replacing sex with time spent together that is about being fully present without distractions. Intimacy is created through genuine time together, not for the purpose of something else like an activity with or for the kids, or talking about who's going to take care of the bills. It is time spent enjoying each other through having fun together and even being silly together. Learn more about your wife, laugh with your wife, and embrace and touch her non-sexually. Give your attention and time to her. Many men have said their relationship improved when they were abstinent with their wife because of their choice to abstain.

You don't need to break up or get divorced; however, you need to become aware of the effect the woman in your life may have on you.

If you are abstinent with a dating partner, your lust for her is probably going to be at a very high point. She triggers you, and that trigger often leads to ejaculation in some form or another that is not with her. A break, and time alone, may be necessary. This may be the tough sacrifice you need to make. You also need to teach yourself that there are other good women out there, and that you have options. You are a man, and what is more valuable to you than freedom from yourself? Without this freedom, you cannot fully love a woman; therefore, this freedom is a priority. You can always get back together or find someone else. The belief that she is the one for you makes you weak and needy. There is no such thing as "the one."

The truth is that men need relationships and some form of intimacy. A common trigger is the imbalance of a romantic relationship without any friendships. Just as with other imbalances, this can make it much harder to recover. While recovering, it is important to make friends and spend time with friends, especially other men. Fill the need for community and relationship. You can work on your communication skills; however, men connect well by doing things rather than by talking about things. Try to stay away from women, especially those who trigger you. Join a community or a club. Going out and meeting people can be hard, especially when you don't have a current friend group. However, putting yourself out there is super important.

MAINTAIN YOUR RECOVERY

Even after you've successfully prevented yourself from sexual release for a period of time, you will still want to entertain thoughts that trigger your mind. If you're not ejaculating, isn't that recovering? Not necessarily. Lustful thoughts will provoke your impulsive triggers, and you will still be affected by them. A lust hangover is when you engage with a lust mentality, or physically, and, as a result, feel extra triggered and aroused for the next day or two. You may not have the intent to fap or ejaculate in some other way, but when you feed your triggers, you increase the uncontrollable urge for it. Do not play with the fire of lust; you will get burned. Whether that is using your imagination in your thoughts, intently baiting yourself with sex to feel the triggers, or flirting, for lustful reasons—all of these are fire. The imagination is the powerhouse area for your triggers. Lustful thoughts will come; however, it is up to you to dismiss them or engage them. Acknowledge your thoughts, but redirect them into prayers, or just let them go. You will get better at this with practice.

You must continue to make the decision for freedom. The beginning can be the hardest, but it must be maintained. After recovering for months, or even years, it is hard to believe you can fall back into your overpowering habit. Men can fall back into their impulsive habits worse than before. There is no such thing as the occasional relapse. You need to continue to live a life of habits that encourage the strength to continue recovery. After the first transformation, the change must be sustained and continued. A muscle that isn't exercised gets weaker.

You will have to figure out what you consistently need so you stay in recovery. Choose some of the habits that have helped you through recovery and continue to practice those habits. Some men who have recovered for several years will still meet with other men to keep them accountable, just like they did when they were in the beginning stages of recovery. Do something, daily or weekly, to keep the spirit of conviction alive. Remember that your impulse will seem, at times, like it might be easier to overcome; however, it is always there. It is ready and willing to express itself through your life and/or through sex. Sex is just the natural go-to for your impulsive energy. It may get easier, but it never gets easy.

Keep a healthy balance of your mind. Do not act out and chase the desire, whether that be with women or sexual stimuli; however, do not entirely deny those sexual desires. Be in the middle, the average of the two. Continue to build a healthy, more balanced life. Your impulse is always there. It is always ready for the imbalance of life. It is always there for you to grab onto when every good and wholesome emotional attachment fails.

YOUR WHY

When in pain, your *why* is easy to remember. Post-nut clarity lets you see more clearly your reasons for recovery. Men don't automatically feel that clear conviction, especially the feeling of regret and shame after ejaculation. Thoughts and emotions swing and shift. We don't forget our why; we just think much less about it. When our brain is flooded with the urge for action through our impulse, it's hard to stay focused. You know you will regret it, but in the moment, you don't care. Your desire for the bliss and ecstasy of your impulse is distracting and convincing you. Even if you truly try to focus on your *why*, it is difficult, and most of the time this may not help much. That's why your *why* needs to be super clear. The strongest why is never discovered in the moment but instead through deep self-reflection and contemplation. A why with no deep meaning will have a hard time going up against the strong, persevering desire of your impulse.

You must find new reasons as well as ongoing convictions about your old reasons. Never get hung up on finding your perfect why. Don't delay your journey because you are uncertain about it; do it because it's good for you! Along the journey you may discover new reasons for overcoming your impulse. Use them and motivate yourself through them. Use your imagination and access your desires and fears to figure out a strong reason for succeeding as well as for not failing.

You must make your actions make sense in your mind. This is continual self-convincing of your why. Ask yourself: what will make you believe without a doubt that this is the right thing to do? The only reason men still fall is because there is a little space where doubt and lack of conviction exist. It is your job to eliminate that doubt as much as possible. You don't just suddenly become convincing, but it happens through deep reflection and contemplation. **Make time for contem-**

plation at least once a week, whether that is through journaling, spending time in deep thought, or discussion. Nobody is going to convince you but yourself. Put this into who you want to be as a man. Your mission and beliefs in life should (indirectly) make it obvious that you are not a man of sexual waste.

It's easy to think that you can stop yourself, but you must realize it is not a thought that needs to change but that *you* need to change. Your current self just failed and will continue to fail. You need to make change. A lasting change. You need to root your decision in something real. When your identity changes, your habits change.

YOU NEED TO ROOT YOUR DECISION IN SOMETHING REAL. WHEN YOUR IDENTITY CHANGES, YOUR HABITS CHANGE.

Our identity is formed by our parents, friends, environment, memories, and what we have done. It is formed by real things and our interpretation of them. Genuine change typically happens slowly—unless something radical happens. Don't expect change when there is nothing to show for it.

Fifteen

Redirection

Every good man is a bad man underneath.

First, sexual redirection is using the same energy that stimulates attraction and ejaculation and turning it into a gift to the world. It's taking that energy and giving it to the universe by sharing your best gifts to find true fulfillment and maximizing your capacity to produce.

On this journey you will become more and more aware of your impulse. You will learn to be in tune with your sexual power, just like a diabetic who can notice whether his blood sugar is too high or low. You can become just as aware of your sexual urges so you can control and redirect them. As men, you feel the power of your impulse, the unstoppable energy and focus that demands sex and demands it *now*. The energy will feel constant. This is not hopeless. You cannot get rid of energy. You can only redirect it.

You need to give this energy a chance. Most men don't know how to cultivate their sexual energy, so they use it and deplete themselves of it. Most men have very little sexual energy because they get rid of it every time they have some. You must teach your body and mind to utilize this power by embracing the surge of energy it gives you. Redirect it from your genitals into your body by taking the focus off of your sexual pleasure, breathing the energy from your genitals into your body, and letting it circulate. Sit with it for a second. Let it enlighten you and fill you with creativity, energy, and alertness. Regulate this power so you will have it at your disposal for use.

All redirection does is put the intense power and energy of your sexual impulse into something more productive. You will begin to utilize it in your everyday life as well as in your goals, tasks, and hobbies. I will teach you tangible ways to utilize this energy; however, you can learn so much from just acknowledging it. It will be like learning how to walk. You will have to experience it and feel it yourself. The first step is to have an awareness of it. Sit with it. Feel it. Notice its patterns and capacity for energy.

To be effective in redirecting this power, you must be able to contain and control it. You have probably had experiences where it has controlled you and even seemed to force you into depleting yourself. I want you to notice its highest intensity points during your day. I want you to recall the last time you completely depleted yourself by relapsing several times. Notice how you won't feel the same urge or desire to continue to relapse. That same desire and drive won't come back instantly, but instead may take several days to fully recharge. The longer you wait, the more you will feel its intensity and the stronger it will be. Can you recall a time when you did not fully deplete yourself and only relapsed once or twice? You may have noticed the difference in the impulsive intensity, that there was still some of it remaining. You may have also noticed that when you relapse, a lesser amount of the energy that could have made you relapse a few more times didn't entirely go away but seemed to sort of linger and grow. (You notice this, especially, when you have more of an urge to relapse much sooner than when you fully depleted yourself the first time.) Most men have naturally noticed this without thinking about it as something with a capacity. Most men, when trying to recover, automatically fully deplete themselves when they relapse once so they can start "strong" without having the same intense urge the next few days.

All highly sexed men recharge their sexual power over time after depleting themselves. Some do so faster than others. As you get older, you will still have this sexual power; however, it will naturally take more time to recharge.

Again, think like the diabetic, who knows exactly how low or high his blood sugar is. I'm going to use percentages to make this tangible to understand. Don't let your sexual energy exceed 90 percent. Zero percent is when you are completely depleted, and 100 percent is when you are at your max capacity of sexual energy. In reality, you may never get to a complete 0 percent or 100 percent, but at somewhere around 0 percent your sexual tension seems to be nonexistent. You usually will be in a very indifferent state. When you are around 100 percent, you feel a *strong* tension. You feel driven, hyper-focused, and hungry for some type of action. Sometimes you can feel ready to explode, and this leads to a mental anxiety that inclines you to act.

Once you become more aware of your sexual energy, you'll be able to tell when it is building up. Some early signs are noticing yourself anticipating sexual release. You are being triggered more than usual. You are engaging in triggering *thoughts* more than usual. The tension in your body is higher than normal.

The problem with your sexual energy getting close to 100 percent is that you become very sensitive to things, especially your impulsive triggers. When your sexual energy is that high, it's very much like it is ready to explode uncontrollably and release massive amounts. You want to avoid letting your sexual energy reach this high.

To control your sexual energy, you must regulate it. Keep it at less than 90 percent. You must use it and let it settle. Whenever you feel your sexual energy getting close to 90 percent, it is time to act on it and lower it. First, you must understand the nature of your sexual power. Even though it recharges, it has a wave-like nature where it can automatically settle down and express itself over a period of time. You may sometimes notice, if you are occupied, that it begins to settle with time. However, you can move it in this direction yourself, and to be able to do so is very important.

One way to express it is through exercise, preferably exercise that is explosive and aggressive. This type of exercise emulates the natural exertion your impulse tends to cause you to use. You are redirecting that impulsive energy and focusing it into a workout rather than sex. It is only over time and practice that you get better and better at redirecting it. You will notice the energy and increased ability to exert this energy during your workouts. It is like a natural pre-workout. After the workout you will notice decreased sexual tension in your body. It may not get rid of the desire to relapse entirely, but it will get rid of the almost unstoppable and uncontrollable sexual intensity you had before. Sports are a great way to use this energy. They involve and fulfill the natural desires of your sexual energy, like action, aggression, and competitiveness. Wrestle, run, fight, compete, and emulate the expression you feel during sex. Emulate the power.

Create new habits that get you to find the same energy and release as ejaculation, just not through ejaculation. Ejaculation can be like a fight for release, freedom, or achievement. It can be used to experience the edge. To stretch ourselves beyond what we thought we were capable of. No man wants sex to be the same, but he wants it to be more than before. The goal is to experience the tension of life and break through the resistance into freedom. Just like how, when playing a sport, you are competing against your opponent with the goal of winning. The goal is to break through the defense so you can score. To break through tension and stress and succeed, bringing relief and ecstasy.

The second way to express and deflate your tension is through slower exertion. This can take more time than the first one; however, you will calm down your energy by letting the impulse/desire settle into your body. You will let the wave of sexual energy pass through, just like "fevering it out." Choose an easy activity. The way sexual power seems to exert itself is mainly through physical stress and not mental stress. Mental stress seems to provoke your desire for sex. You can go for a walk, do a relaxing activity, meditate, and even take a nap. It's not so much about the quick exertion but allowing the sexual energy to move through your body. It is being expressed, just not quickly or with high impact. Ride the wave of the intensity and let it settle. Let it come and go because, if you interfere, it will affect you by causing some kind of anxiety or even arousing you. Express the sexual energy by using it and letting it express itself through magnifying your body by the way you feel. Through your alertness and the circulation of this energy, it will make you feel alive.

LET IT INSPIRE YOU

Redirection is like surfing, mastering the powerful energy of the waves; like feeling, through the rise and the fall of your impulse, without losing focus but adjusting when necessary to keep the balance, and thus riding the wave of your impulse.

After you have fully charged (see fully charge, in chapter 3 of this book) your sexual energy following a state of depletion, you will feel the surge of your impulse come and go. This is energy. When the energy fills your body, the learned association with its feelings is sexual arousal. It is up to you to react to the feelings as you choose. It can also bring feelings of inspiration, creativity, aliveness, and ambition. It may bring anxiety, sometimes positive, sometimes negative. However, it is up to you to interpret the tendencies and decide whether you should use this urge for relaxing or for more intense activities. Once you master and utilize the onset of this energy, you begin to recognize that when it comes, it won't be around for long.

If you want control and positive direction for the sexual energy, let it inspire you. When inspired, magnify it by engaging with it and letting it expand. Use this time to create and enjoy life. Hone in your inspiration by acting on it. If you are working on a project, you can still work on it; however, let the energy work through you. Let it enhance your focus and productivity. Let it inspire creativity in you. If you're working out, let the inspired energy help boost your workout intensity and focus. It may inspire you to drop your task and do something else. Let the energy move you. You can use this surge to your advantage, whether that is by letting it inspire you to complete your most stressful tasks, like making your biggest decisions, or simply using the surge to inspire you to do your chores or just clean a room in your house or apartment. This energy will never make you completely lose control because you still have options of how to express the energy; however, be open-minded to its suggestions.

(The surge reminds me of what it is like when your dog gets what some call the zoomies. Zoomies is a term for dogs when they get a crazy look in their eyes, tuck their butt, and start vigorously running wild laps around your house or yard. It has been referred to as "zoomies," "crazy eights," "midnight madness," and "demon possession." Nobody knows the cause; however, dogs seem to do this so they can alleviate stress or release pent-up energy.)

Embrace and amplify your arousal not just through your genitalia but to your whole body. Let it affect you in the most unrestrained ways. Let it fly free in the feeling and movements of your body. Enjoy its rambunctious attitude, and let it fully enlighten your body and mind. Dance your heart out, yell at the top of your lungs, beat your chest like you are king of the world. Let it refresh and remind you of the gift of life. Connect with your humanity and the deepest and most impactful part of you as a man.

In this moment, work out intensely. Grunt from the deepest part of you. Let the slavery of your impulse express its freedom. Freedom without any hesitation or holding back. Freedom is nothing if we do not use it. Express it and show gratitude for it.

When encountering a beautiful woman who you find attractive through the looks of her body or even her personality, you begin to automatically direct energy to your brain and genitals with fantasies and lustful thoughts. You have probably felt a strong attraction for one or many women in your life. An attraction that is captivating and intoxicating. Attraction can bring out great inspiration in men. Inspiration for action and creation in the arts or by pursuing ambitious goals. The source of creativity for many men has been stimulated by women, as can be seen through a direct expression of their music and art. Most creative men will admit that their inspiration came from women. Many men, however, will quickly deplete this energy through some sort of poor stimulation or even ejaculation.

You must let your impulse do its thing. You may feel unproductive when taking time to redirect your energy with daily activities, as well as using energy to avoid triggers. This may feel uncomfortable if you are not used to it. If you were to relapse, you would have the illusion of doing so allowing you to remain "productive." When experiencing a feeling of discomfort from "wasting" time, sit with it a little longer. Let your impulse do its work in you. Your impulse can inspire you to do tasks in an hour when originally they would take a day. The focus and intensity you get from redirecting your energy can turn the last couple hours of a nonproductive day into a very productive one. Your impulse may get you to act on things that would have taken you a week or month to complete. You will quickly learn that there will be times you need to back off from working and times you can't help yourself from getting things done.

To redirect this energy, use your breathing to shift the energy from your mind and genitalia to your body. Breathe and let it circulate, giving new life to every cell. Feel the energy and be present to let it inspire you to action. Seek how you can give and express this energy for the greater good. Let it kick-start you to action. Let it inspire your imagination.

ACT ON IT

Don't desire or wish that your impulse is gone. Rather, wish that you had more control over it. You master your impulse when it neither sways nor moves you, when you fully embrace the powerful intensity and are able and even grateful to use it and instill its gifts. You learn to desire the redirection of it.

After beginning the process of abstaining, men notice the difference in their energy levels. They feel more energetic and stronger, and they have more endurance.

The changing of the mind also occurs, usually automatically and quite quickly, when you start abstaining from your impulse. You will instantly have more time and energy, and the motives of your mind and the way you see things will change.

When your mind isn't looking for fulfillment through sex, it will need to find fulfillment somewhere else. Men usually notice that they feel more ambitious and have a strong desire to accomplish things. They also may notice an increase in creativity and imagination, urging them to create, perform, and pursue more of these gifts.

Men put a lot of their energy into sexual thoughts. It's okay to feel the attraction and recognize an attraction, but you do not have to deeply engage or invest in those thoughts. The same goes when you have multiple thoughts of ambitious goals. Redirection is having the ability to funnel those thoughts into just a few ambitious goals where you can make a greater investment of your energy without scattering your thoughts as waste. The brain does not automatically interpret good or bad thoughts. It invests energy, and that energy encourages action.

When invested in your purpose and goals, you can let that energy flow without battling to prevent action that you fear you might take. You feel neither exhausted nor unsatisfied by this.

Humans also can be overwhelmed by variety. Variety is good, but too much is exhausting. Less is more, especially when investing in thoughts and ideas. A man who spreads his power too thin cannot effectively use that power. Invest it in a purpose and mission. This will give you meaning, which is more fuel and encouragement for your redirection of power. A man can magnify his power when what he invests it in is a meaningful goal. The fulfillment of this goal will act as a continuous cycle feeding back into your decision to redirect and further magnify your productivity.

Men who are focused on purpose notice an absence of sexual desire. Some men will question if they have erectile dysfunction but find out they do not. This is because their purpose has redirected their sexual energy. Always have a meaningful purpose and mission in your life. As soon as you complete one purpose, find another.

Men have attributes that can be perceived in either positive or negative ways. These attributes are in the biology of men, and men find a way to use them or suppress them. When they are suppressed, men will not function efficiently or feel fulfillment in themselves. These attributes can be used through ways they need to express themselves and meet their needs. Your impulse has been a substitute for action, aggression, ambition, competition, production, and survival. Your impulse has been filling these needs for you, directly or indirectly. You can say the same thing about video games and movies. The human brain can use virtual reality to express these tendencies. Video games, movies, and especially sex are all ways to express and fill these needs.

These ways of expression, and the use of internal instincts and motives, are shallow and rarely make a man feel truly fulfilled. If a man tells you he is truly fulfilled by his video game achievements, a football game-watching streak, or a porno collection, wait until his ego dies and ask him the same question again.

If you are stressed and have tension building up, go to your car where no one can hear you and yell as loud as you can; vigorously do sprints; or dance, releasing and expressing the tension. You will notice yourself feeling less tense than before. Now think about if you just let that stress build and build without releasing it. What will probably happen is you will find a way to release it whether you want to or not. If stressed enough, you may feel like you are forced to release energy through lashing out at someone or just losing your temper. As humans, we develop habits, usually subconsciously, to release mental and sexual tension. What's important is exactly how we release the tension. Physical and emotional expression is a form of release. We feel better when we express and find fulfillment through it, whether that is temporary unhealthy fulfillment or more lasting healthy fulfillment.

Take away someone's habits of expression and they will find other forms of expression. Take away a child's toy, and sooner or later the child will find something else to play with. The only difference is that your new ways of expressing these needs are, hopefully, more fulfilling than the old ways, as well as more useful and productive ways to spend time and release tension.

Men are less likely to feel lazy, for they are not depleted and still seek to fulfill their needs. They will have the right kind of ambition.

They are more likely to have a genuine excitement about other activities. They are filled with the life of their impulse.

Your impulse has the power to make rash decisions, act quickly, and exert strength and conviction. People may say your impulse is dangerous. It can be dangerous; however, a great man cannot be great unless he starts with the potential to be great. This potential to be good is also the potential to be evil. Power is neither good nor evil; it is only your morals that will direct it. Don't be afraid of the strength even though you know you are capable of major damage. Don't forget it is the lukewarm who God spits out (Revelation chapter 3 in the Bible). It is because you have nothing to work with when you are lukewarm. Remember that time you decided to act on your impulse? Not just a wishy-washy decision, but the decision that made you turn abruptly and storm toward action? Remember your sexual climax. Notice the unstoppable focus, the endurance of your intent, and the strength given to your passionate feelings. If a man can control these qualities, let alone redirect some of them, this man is truly powerful.

> *"You should be a monster. An absolute monster.*
> *And then you should learn how to control it."*
> –JORDAN PETERSON

Embrace your impulsive power. You feel the strength and the tension behind it. The ability to focus and do what is on your heart even if it is difficult. Notice the last time you ejaculated: the intensity and focus you used to simulate tension and release it to great relief and satisfaction. Think about the many times you have decided not to engage in sexual activity, and yet it was like you were overtaken by a powerful force that made the decision to engage in it anyway (with unstoppable conviction in the moment). Your impulse is demonstrating the fearless decision to engage or disengage, the strength to take massive action, and the laser-like focus to stick to this action all the way through.

Your impulse is like a loaded gun; use it to your advantage.

Highly sexed men have both the gift and curse of their impulse. When they use it as a gift it can transform their life. The nature of this impulse is demonstrated in the confident decisions a leader makes when everybody else is afraid and indecisive. This is demonstrated in the man who loses his marriage and his kids but takes action to restart his life by picking up new hobbies, setting new goals, and fearlessly trudging ahead to create a better life for himself. This is also demonstrated in the man who makes the fearless decision to go off to war even when it is dangerous and he might lose his life. The man who physically and passionately fights another man or animal to defend others. The man willing to sacrifice his life for what he believes no matter the loss or pain. And the man who keeps his word, sticks to the mission, and perseveres through challenges and obstacles. These men know there is no other way toward true peace and fulfillment. This is what it takes to be powerful and redirect that power toward good.

> THE NATURE OF THIS IMPULSE IS DEMONSTRATED IN THE CONFIDENT DECISIONS A LEADER MAKES WHEN EVERYBODY ELSE IS AFRAID AND INDECISIVE.

Men have demonstrated the use of this power throughout history. They have changed lives and changed the world. The deep yearning and dissatisfaction you feel inside as a man isn't nothing. It's a portal of power ready to be released into a meaningful life. Women have their own deep feminine gifts; however, men are the ones who fight the wars, decide on the course of their country, sacrifice their lives, and invent and create solutions to problems. It is not just that men do these things, but that they are inspired and have a longing to do these things. This is innately related to the nature of men. The need to produce and protect is a built-in desire.

Men desire to fight, to witness violence, and to test their strength and the strength of their peers. They may desire to be in war and face a deadly challenge. If they do not express it, they admire it. It is the power of the impulse wanting to release and express itself. It can make a bad man enhance his ability to do bad, but it can also make a good man enhance his ability to do good.

This is demonstrated in the decisions we make, the massive actions we take, and the unstoppable motivation and focus we have.

The uncontrollable power to urgently engage in sexual activity is just like—we could even say it "emulates" —your ability to disregard all fear and make a necessary decision. Your intense and unstoppable concentration during sexual activity emulates your ability to stick to your guns and be firm in your belief without swaying from your truth, and to go through until the end of the mission. Last, the blissful and powerful act of ejaculation emulates your fulfillment in the completion of a mission. The satisfaction of giving to the world, achieving the goal, and finding a sense of freedom.

> THIS IS DEMONSTRATED IN THE DECISIONS WE MAKE, THE MASSIVE ACTIONS WE TAKE, AND THE UNSTOPPABLE MOTIVATION AND FOCUS WE HAVE.

The nature of your impulse is to manipulate your thoughts, to be ever-present and enduring, to take massive uncontrollable action, and to persevere with laser focus until ejaculation. These are not bad qualities unless used in the wrong context. Let your impulse drive you when it is necessary. Let it manipulate your mind when you're doing the right thing. Let it be enduring and present when you're working on creating a goal, let it take massive action when you need to make a decision, and let it help you to persevere and keep focused when you need to complete a mission. Express it, but in a way that helps you. Let it loose. You are now aware that you are the owner of an "animal," a beast. You need to let it run around the yard and do its thing, or it will cause trouble. Let it run free, but put its muzzle and leash on when necessary. Take care of it and take care of yourself. It is a deep part of you, and it does you no good not to be aware of it and its nature.

SEX BECOMES MORE APPRECIATED

Action reinforces new beliefs. Your habits train your mind. After years and years of hookups and weekly porn, the brain changes.

When you abstain, sex becomes more of a gift than a priority. You no longer need it to still enjoy it. The choice you make to engage in sex becomes more authentic. What is the value of sex when you give it out for free? When abstaining, women become more personable and human to you. Before it wasn't about the person or the relationship. It was about the feeling and need to satisfy your impulse. The woman was merely a stepping-stone to get you to where you "needed to be."

WHEN YOU START EXPRESSING YOUR NEED INTO SOMETHING PRODUCTIVE, YOUR LIFE BECOMES MORE VALUABLE. YOU ARE AN ASSET TO THE WORLD INSTEAD OF A LIABILITY THAT NEEDS SLEEP, FOOD, AND PORN.

Life becomes more meaningful. When you start expressing your need into something productive, your life becomes more valuable. You are an asset to the world instead of a liability that needs sleep, food, and porn. Everything else becomes inherently more valuable to you. You see the world differently because you can add to it. You have real and actual control over your life. It has been your playground; you just have to get yourself unstuck from the mud. You may not find how to express your gifts to the world just yet, but you are now available to do so. Ready yourself to give your gifts when the opportunity arises. You are a free man who broke up with his demanding relationship with sex.

WAYS TO LIVE THIS REDIRECTION

Spread out your sexual energy. Redirection doesn't mean you have to become a macho hyper-aggressive man but a man who uses more of his power in the ways he chooses. Yes, you can still redirect this power into becoming aggressive and assertive, but this is not required to overcome and redirect your impulse.

What you focus on and choose to invest your energy in is redirecting your power. You already have some of this power, even as a depleted man. The difference between the depleted and the nondepleted man is the difference in potential power. The man is the director of his own power, but the amount and magnification of that power can change and transform his life. The depleted man automatically has less of a handle on his power, and the little power that he directs is deflated. When you control your impulse by not depleting yourself through sex, you will automatically have better control over the redirection of it.

When you refuse to deplete yourself and are present with charged sexual power, you will naturally start to redirect it. You begin to let it influence you. This power exists and must go somewhere. Even if you do nothing, you are letting it manifest itself in your body and mind, creating new and influencing emotions, feelings, and vigor that can get you to act. The more control you have over your impulse, the better you will be able to redirect the energy and focus you would use for sex into your life and work.

You can redirect this energy in different ways. It's common to picture this sexual energy as passion and aggression, usually by working out, accomplishing tasks quickly, and making hasty decisions. This way of expression probably comes to mind because you can feel this type of expression deep in your core as a man. Men desire to be physical, to act and move with force. Men may fulfill this desire by getting into sports, wrestling with their friends, and other things of this nature. Like the macho man, the man redirecting his sexual energy expresses a good amount of his sexual energy through his body.

A different expression of sexual energy is that of the monk. You may automatically think this man is like the depleted, married man who is calm and sedated, but he is not. The monk may look calm physically, but mentally and spiritually he is alive and enlightened. His sexual energy is directed into his ability to focus. His ambition from his sexual energy is expressed in his desire for spiritual achievement.

So the monk is calm but redirects his power—which is still there—toward a deeper meaningful life in the spiritual world. Most men regularly deplete themselves and are often exhausted of sexual power. The monk and the depleted man may both appear to be sedated on the outside, but the level of intention they give to their daily lives is entirely different. A depleted man has less meaning in his life than he would have as a sexually charged man. The depleted man is more careless and unintentional than he would be otherwise. It is not about the intent and care you give everything but what you specifically choose to invest your power in. The monk may not care about food, sports, or other matters in this world, but he puts his care and intent into his spiritual life and journey, therefore magnifying the care and intent for it. He doesn't share his opinions with the world, but if you talk to him about his spiritual life, he will have a strong one, and it will mean everything to him. In contrast, the depleted man may be opinionless or express his opinions and beliefs, but he will do nothing about them because they do not truly mean anything to him.

Be aware that sexual expression isn't the only way to deplete yourself of sexual power. No man will consciously choose to deplete himself of his power without hesitation. This man is, rather, allowing life to deplete him of it. It is the unfulfilling "meaning" he has in his life, or the lack of meaning. Depletion is when you choose to give your time, energy, and intent toward things you don't believe in or care about. It is having a hesitation to give, and yet giving anyway. Your impulsive power is a gift, and when it is not given genuinely, it destroys rather than creates. Instead of your gifts enlightening you, you are drained of power.

A man's sexual impulse becomes his main source of meaning. You may not think so, but you act so. Your impulse, just like the sexual time and energy you put toward nothing you truly believe in, leaves you depleted. An example of this is porn, or careless promiscuous sex, and how either can make you feel depleted right away. Other common ways of depleting yourself are giving your time and energy to your work, culture, and even your wife. They are all influencing you to do things you don't deeply believe in. When you don't have your own convictions about what you should do or believe in, you will be given beliefs and convictions by the culture and those around you. When you are indecisive about something, it is usually your subconscious telling you that it may not be worth your power and should be looked into.

Don't give your power to something you are not convicted about. Make those boundaries so you are not depleted. Your energy must flow, but let it flow into something that rejuvenates you—or at least doesn't exhaust you of power. It is going to be about choosing your convictions; however, starting with your non-convictions and what you are not willing to invest your time and energy in is very important. Sometimes, in order to choose your convictions, things start with consciously choosing your non-convictions and figuring out how to cut off your portal of power into that area. If you know what you want to invest your power in, great, but sometimes you don't know, and the only and best thing for you is to prepare yourself to be accessible to the next opportunity to invest this power.

Married men, even in a sexless marriage, can still be depleted of this power by their wives. It is common to see a man's wife tell him to do things he doesn't believe in; however, he does them anyway because he feels obligated to. He is enslaved to someone else's beliefs and ideas and are acting against his own intuition. Most men, when looking inward, don't have their own strong beliefs in the first place. You may not believe in something, but it is the acting and allowing that depletes you of power.

For example, a man may feel obligated to do things for his wife even when, deep down, he doesn't want to, and maybe the people who are surrounding and influencing him that he should are right. However, it is not hopeless for the man. In these cases, someone who is responsible would take it upon himself to form his own beliefs and convictions so he knows if he should or should not be obligated to serve his wife, and why. The responsible man would seek to make his own beliefs, whether those are in agreement or contrary to the beliefs of others. It is up to him to use reason and logic to form his beliefs. The depleted married man and the nondepleted married man can do the same "obligations" for his wife day in and day out. One man is exhausted and depressed because he doesn't believe and truly know why he is doing these things for his wife, and the other is refreshed and rejuvenated because he has formed his own beliefs and knows why he needs to fulfill his obligations for his wife. Same task, different convictions. One man can be doing the right thing but be unsatisfied because he doesn't know why he is doing it.

If your family, wife, or friends work hard to convince you to "believe in" something, it is up to you to truly decide on that belief or not, especially if it requires your action and cooperation. A nondepleted man does his work genuinely because he chooses to. Yes, maybe his wife and parents would make him take an action, which would deplete him because it would enslave him to do so. Rather, he came up with his own reasons to do it himself, and it freed him because he is no longer doing it out of obligation but through genuine belief. It is an

PEOPLE ARE MORE INVESTED IN SOMETHING WHEN IT IS THEIR CHOICE.

obligation because he says it is an obligation. People are more invested in something when it is their choice.

Until an authentic decision is made, no man is truly free if he doesn't make those beliefs and traditions his own. Leave others the benefit of the doubt until proven otherwise. Whether rejecting or accepting a personal belief, be sure to search thoroughly whether it makes sense, and do so with an open mind and unbiased heart. If worse comes to worst, you can respectfully disagree; however, the self-seeking will make you genuine and honest, which are admirable traits no matter who you are. Your personal freedom is your responsibility, and it is up to you to question the beliefs bestowed on you, not so you can disrespect them, but so you can genuinely agree (or disagree) with them. Genuine action has a great impact no matter how small the task.

Men in today's culture speak about settling down. The idea of settling down usually comes from him wanting to rejuvenate himself because he is exhausted, and something is depleting him of his power. For a man who redirects his power, settling down should never be about calming down but about reinvesting his power into something else meaningful and rejuvenating. Even though a man's sex drive may decrease with age, he still has the same impulsive power he used to; therefore, he still has the ability, and urge, to give his power to the world in a rejuvenating way. The sexual drive is built to give life both psychologically and physically. Most men are happy and healthy when they choose to work after retirement. Working is what men do. It is how they give and find satisfaction. It is common for men to die not long after living with no real purpose, following retirement; this is because mission and meaning are essential to a man's life. Once you cut off your mission, you start to deteriorate in both mind and body, just like how a car needs to be run for the battery to recharge. Men need to work to be healthier.

Your imagination is stimulated through your impulse. Think of how your impulse acts: always looking for new sexual experiences, and when doing so, it has an imagination that is vibrant and creative.

Take that vibrant creativity and transfer it from your impulse to your work and life. You have a natural tendency to seek things that are new and different. This refreshes and stimulates you, just like how a different sexual experience stimulates your arousal. When you know everything and what is going to happen, you become bored and depressed; however, the excitement of variety can enliven and even cure you. You are creative, and your mind seeks to be creative. When we use our creativity toward our sexual impulse, it limits the excitement and creativity toward other things, redirecting its flow into what matters in life. Let it lighten you up and fill your work and life with creativity. Your impulse has demonstrated its power to create and express, but it is never a fulfilled creation, or expression, until it is redirected into something truly meaningful. Once you move this creativity away from your impulsive desire, you give it access to your life and what really matters to you. Your imagination can run free in a new and refreshing way.

In the same way that you might have looked for the right sex position or a porn video to please your impulse, do precisely the same with your creative mind. Your impulsive mind will find satisfaction in creativity, and that will excite you. This is a form of impulsive release. Let the creativity flow through a new channel. Let its power enhance your abilities. Get lost in your art. Your strong impulse is indirectly telling you to take a break from your current task, and that you need an activity that is both spontaneous and freeing. Build, paint, or otherwise create with a spontaneous, free mind, and you will get lost to the point that your impulse seems to be satisfied and doesn't disturb you. Your impulse is expressing its power through your creativity, and it is up to you to let it flow. Follow your impulse into its creativity. Read its signs. It's like a dog on a leash; every once in a while you will let it roam free and run a bit wild. Sometimes that dog will dig up the treasure you wanted but never expected. Start playing with your creative impulse. Try writing, painting, or music, and let your impulse connect to one of these arts.

The tension you feel from your sexual impulse is being filled up with its pressure to be released. This pressure is energy meant to be a gift to the world. Men are built to give psychologically and physically. Look at the male body, which is built to give its seed. It isn't empty inside, nor does it have a womb to receive seed like the female body. Instead, it is made to recharge and give from within. Men are naturally designed to constantly fill up with pressure and tension. This is why they desire, in one sense, emptiness. To release this pressure and give it away. It is a cycle of constant constraint and freedom. Tension and release.

Men will naturally desire to seek freedom physically, emotionally, and spiritually, whether that is to free themselves from the defense when playing a sport, or from the constraint and control of an opponent in war. Men desire to overcome a challenge, to be held back by nothing. To seek fears and obstacles, to overcome them and break through. Healthy men with no tension, either physically, emotionally, or spiritually, will naturally seek tension. Once they have it, their goal is to release it. And the cycle repeats itself.

The nature of your impulse is to win, break through barriers, discover, and feel the ecstasy of freedom. It emulates the tension built in sex and released in ejaculation. If you don't express it periodically, it will find a way to express itself.

You can see actual power in the impulse through watching other highly sexed men. They tend toward action, aggression, ambition, competition, and production because of this search for tension and freedom. If they do not express these tendencies, they feel as if they have to. To physically fight or beat the next video game level is an example of this expression. They will do this even if it is in an unhealthy and unrefreshing way. Highly sexed men who seem more depleted, calm, and sedate than other men are over-depleting themselves in ways that are not rejuvenating. They find some sort of expression, usually in the form of pornography, video games, sex, or through some other means.

Others, and the culture, fear and despise these inclinations because of the power behind them. The power to destroy but also to reconstruct. Own these dark and dangerous tendencies you have. Do not fear them but explore them. Do not try to reject them but find a place for them. Redirect them and use them as a gift. Express the darkest parts of you and form a new, healthy alliance with them. Make this new identity a gift to yourself and the world.

It is natural to express these attributes. It just matters how you do it so they are healthy and refreshing. When you are stressed, uncertain, sexually charged, or angry you can either direct those feelings and energy toward masturbation—or go to the gym, develop yourself, and/or otherwise take massive action toward your goals.

Men who express themselves honestly and vulnerably during sex express aggression and assertiveness. . . .

David Deida says, in *The Way of the Superior Man* (chapter 36):

"The difference between rape and ravishment is love."

MINDSET

A convicted mind is an unstoppable mind, whether for good or for bad. Redirect your focus to a focus that supports your mission. Remind yourself of the transformation and benefits of your recovery.

Your impulse can be not only your source of power but your greatest teacher. Any teacher may teach you an important lesson, but it is the excellent ones who instill this lesson into your character. These lessons change us for the better. Your recovery teaches you through experience. Experience is like a mental tattoo. A scar that fades but is always there. Rather than just the acquiring of knowledge, it turns into lessons that are much more personal and profound.

One of the greatest lessons your impulse can teach you is to be in the now. When you embrace the moment and fully live in the present, looking back will be an experience full of memories and not one of regrets. You will have to face the constant tension created by your sexual energy. If you try to ignore it in the present moment, you will fail. You will be reminded often of your impulse and its never-exhausted push for expression. Your impulse is a parallel to the constant struggle and wrestles of life. It is so easy to fall into the trap of believing that reaching one goal will make you happy. If you ask other men, they will say they don't live by this concept, but watch their actions, and you will see that most men live as though they are betting everything on one goal. They exhaust themselves with the belief that accomplishment will grant them rest and that they'll be fulfilled for the rest of their days. These men are like dogs chasing their own tails, and they are getting exhausted by doing so. Your impulse reminds you of the constant wrestle, and it also reminds you to embrace it because that is the best way to combat it. You cannot run away from it, so you either cave to it or magnify it. Let your impulse teach you to live in the moment and to know no end to your missions, to live each one out by maximizing them through truly giving. Use the impulse to strengthen your talents so you can give to the world and others. Seek fulfillment through what you are doing and not through the destination/end goal of "where" you are seeking to make it to.

ONE OF THE GREATEST LESSONS YOUR IMPULSE CAN TEACH YOU IS TO BE IN THE NOW. WHEN YOU EMBRACE THE MOMENT AND FULLY LIVE IN THE PRESENT, LOOKING BACK WILL BE AN EXPERIENCE FULL OF MEMORIES AND NOT ONE OF REGRETS.

It can teach you how to live in the moment and find joy through relaxing in that moment. Your impulse can force you to relax, especially when you're feeling the tension building from when you don't relax.

It can teach you to be free of all other worries because you must prioritize when you are recovering. You can't waste energy on other worries because you are focused on more important goals. When you lose focus on recovering, you will fail. You cannot afford to give a care about anything else. Such a feeling is beautiful. It allows you to let go of other worries because you know you have to in order to succeed. It will bring out the fiercest part of you and teach you how to control it. For you to say a committed yes to your recovery, you have to say no to everything else that is not recovery and mean it. You will need the courage to rock the boat of life.

Why does a man get hooked on sex in the first place? It is the seeking of satisfaction, freedom, and fulfillment. Sometimes it can seem like it's just to relieve the tension. However, men use sex to fill their lives and needs, and yet they find it very shallow and unsatisfying. It deceives through promising fulfillment and yet never meets those needs and just makes you hungrier for more. This makes you question your humanity as a man. What is the point? What shall I do? Is fulfillment possible? Yes, but it never lasts. Now, if it never lasts, is it a worthy goal to seek to attain? Most men don't want to ask these questions because they don't want to hear the answers. The truth is that there is no pure and lasting satisfaction in this life. Satisfaction is real, but only tastes of it. Certain things will bring you more satisfaction than others. It's ironic that people usually don't feel satisfied when they are focusing on themselves, but when they are focused on others. They never feel fulfilled when they are taking, but rather giving. The lesson from your sexual desire is the example of the always-giving attitude, the never-ending opportunity to give, and the purpose for your life to keep releasing your gifts. You may rest and refresh, but there is nothing else that will fulfill you like giving.

We can start giving by changing our focus and priorities. Instead of focusing on taking from others, focus on what you can give instead. Instead of using your sexual desire to find satisfaction in yourself, use it to drive you to give pure satisfaction to the world and others.

A fulfilled man is giving the fullest of himself to the world. He gives to the world what he believes it needs.

"The way a man penetrates the world should be the same way he penetrates his woman: not merely for personal gain or pleasure, but to magnify love, openness, and depth."
—DAVID DEIDA

It is freeing to come to the realization that you are truly vulnerable and susceptible to acting out if you don't change *something*. The journey seems difficult and unbearable, but there are gems along the roadside that will change your life. You will obtain a new level of consciousness about yourself and the world. There is something different about acquiring knowledge and learning from experience. Knowledge is on the surface, but experience is engrained in you. You may have many realizations on your recovery journey, and they are all there to help you grow. The first realization you may have is developing new ways to see your impulse. Most men never know the true strength of their impulse, how the impulse makes the mind sick, and the experience of taking positive action when they are uncertain of what to do. By combating our impulse, we feel its strength and test its power, and we become stronger and more resilient because of it.

Your impulse will teach you to act in the face of conflict and uncertainty. Your impulse will trick you with seemingly convincing thoughts and make you lose your certainty. To overcome your impulse, you must teach yourself to act against it. This illusion, this distraction, makes you unable to focus and think clearly, but you will get good at acting on and sticking to what you know is truth. The impulse will be resilient, but you will learn how to be more resilient. There is nothing more inspiring than a man who perseveres in what he knows to be truth and acts in certainty when everything around him and inside him is chaos.

Overcoming your impulse will teach you to be proactive in life. Most of the time you don't relapse because you did something, but because you did nothing. Unlike having the courage to stick up for yourself . . . unlike when you ask a hot girl out . . . instead you make excuses even though you know in your heart you need to act. It is easier to wait until it is too late and ignore that small feeling inside. But we realize it is better to act than not act. We feel less shame when we fail than if we were to never act at all.

> BUT WE REALIZE IT IS BETTER TO ACT THAN NOT ACT. WE FEEL LESS SHAME WHEN WE FAIL THAN IF WE WERE TO NEVER ACT AT ALL.

Your impulse will teach you to continue to work on yourself. It's like fixing an old car that needs restored. You need to replace virtually every part to get it up and running and in good condition. Once it's up and running, it's great! Occasionally you will take it out for a drive, and all of a sudden something will go wrong. Something will always go wrong on your journey, whether you lose conviction or find an unexpected trigger. Back to the car: as long as you maintain and keep fixing it, it will do just fine. But once you stop taking care of your car, it is sure to break down. It has to be maintained. You must have the end in mind.

Sexual power is a gift. Use it or be used by it. When they say, "Idle hands are the devil's workshop," well, this also applies to your impulse. You were meant to work and give, whether that is a humble and meaningless task or not. It's not so much about finding the right work but putting yourself out there to, first, just work; in time, the right tasks will be revealed to you. Choose to use this power before it has an influence on you. Use its influence for good. Your sexual impulse is only as useful to you as your interpretation of it. Instead of watching your impulse urge you toward sex, interpret it as it telling you simply to get off your butt, work out, fix your problems, and pursue a goal.

Men will do anything but acknowledge their obsessive impulse. Nobody wants to acknowledge it fully. Acceptance of it seems like death. Death of your false reality. Pride seems to crawl up on everybody. We seem to slap labels on things, meanings, and dreams, and they can be as far from reality as we want—as long as we keep on tricking ourselves into believing them. The nature of pride is to create beliefs, and if those beliefs become barriers, they need to be knocked down. Our egos may be in the way of admitting we're in the wrong. Since they are our sense of identity, it hurts to knock them down. We feel lonely and lost without an identity. But, to advance in life, we need to build a new one. Your impulse is there to remind you of reality and who you truly are.

Your impulse keeps you accountable to continually surrendering your meaningless wants so you can stay in reality and give to the world more fully. It will teach you to do the humble and simple techniques that actually make a difference. Most men are looking for the prize of recovery to be easy and extraordinary, but sometimes the most extraordinary thing they are looking for is found in the journey—in the thick of the fight. A reward isn't so meaningful to the one who didn't earn it.

You will learn that dependability isn't the answer. You will never find the right relationship. Marriage isn't the solution, fellows. It is best to overcome your impulse before you are married. It is best to learn how to swim before you are thrown into water. Become independent because you are the only earthly being you can truly depend on. All else is out of your control, and all else will perish.

Control won't come naturally to a reactive man. Control is learned and will be earned by your own strength and through being proactive. You see your impulsive tendencies before they come, and you act on them right away. The best way to learn is through experience. This is a test of your strength, but most importantly, it is a journey. Don't be afraid to fail, nor to "fake it until you make it," especially when it comes to what works. You need to practice the right techniques (many have been mentioned in this chapter, and in earlier chapters) because you know that you should, not because you "feel like it."

Last, this will teach you self-discipline. To *not* rely on sheer will-power because the will . . . is weak. Rather, to put your effort into outsmarting your strong desires. And to train yourself to follow through with your goals despite temptation.

THE BEST WAY TO LEARN IS THROUGH EXPERIENCE. THIS IS A TEST OF YOUR STRENGTH, BUT MOST IMPORTANTLY, IT IS A JOURNEY.

Sixteen

Transformation

Recovery has many benefits. One is that it increases a man's testosterone. During three weeks of no ejaculation, there is already a difference in a man's testosterone level. Increased testosterone alone has multiple benefits. However, there are more benefits men notice from their recovery journey.

RELATIONSHIP BENEFITS

1. Improved relationships

2. Better sexual taste

3. Better connection with another person

4. More naturally attracted to sex

5. Improved healthy sex life

6. Being more respectable (gaining more respect)

7. Better social life

8. Appear more attractive to women; women have told such men they "are different"

9. Deeper and stronger bonds in a relationship

MENTALLY

1. Mental clarity

2. Reduced stress or pressure

3. More relaxed

4. Reduced rage or anger

5. Increased willpower

6. Increased focus and concentration

7. Gain deeper emotion

8. Increased motivation

9. Reduced sexual anxiety

10. Improved confidence

11. Increased self-esteem

12. Emotional balance

13. Greater appreciation for art and beauty

14. A sharper mind

15. Less depression

16. More competitive

17. A better and greater sense of purpose

PHYSICAL

1. Deeper voice

2. More facial hair

3. Clearer skin

4. More energy

5. Better stamina

6. Feeling "more alive"

LIFE/WORK

1. Better work ethic

2. More productive

3. More time to enjoy life

4. Better life achievement

HARNESS YOUR SEXUAL POWER THROUGH ABSTINENCE

When a person is hungry, they look for food. The hungrier they get, the more urgently they search for food. A male's body will automatically produce sexual energy so he can reproduce. Just like when abstaining from sex, you desire, urgently, to look for sex. You become motivated and determined. But now, instead, harness that power and use its motivation and determination toward your goals. It is not only directive but receptive. That is why avoiding your triggers is important. Imagine a magnetic force. As long as you move a magnet toward another magnet of your choice, you can tap into its magnetic pull—but it also has to be clear of any other magnet that will interfere with the pull. The other magnets represent triggers that deter you from your goals. It's up to you to be smart and aware of your surroundings as well as strong enough when caught by the other magnetic pull to move your magnet away and reposition it.

EVERYTHING WILL BECOME MUCH CLEARER

"Sobriety makes you feel better;
you feel anger better and resentment better."
–Unknown

The truth is all your feelings are enhanced, even the positive ones. You have been numbed by depletion, and now you get to feel the strength of freedom. Unproductive release of your sexual energy was just a cover-up for true expression. Emotions arise that were there all along but could not express themselves. Depletion is a cover-up for both the joyful and painful emotions. Most men don't notice their underlying ambitions or insecurities because they are blinded by their impulse.

> A HIGHLY SEXED MAN'S SEX DRIVE IS NOT FOR WIMPS. YOU HAVE TO BE FEARLESS AND RELENTLESS. YOU CANNOT BE A PUSHOVER. YOU MUST HAVE THE MINDSET OF A WARRIOR.

Besides all the benefits of recovery, you will be transformed into a stronger man. A highly sexed man's sex drive is not for wimps. You have to be fearless and relentless. You cannot be a push-over. You must have the mindset of a warrior. You must be dangerous, and you must fight dirty. Your recovery pro-cess alone will teach you to be powerful and to fight fearlessly. The inner beast in you will come out. It has to. You will be stressed out, upset, and angry, but it is the beast in you that decides to pull through and fight. You will be knocked off your guard and dazed.

You may momentarily forget why are you in recovery, but it is the true human spirit that keeps swinging and attacking. You will become powerful because recovery will force you to be powerful. A man is as powerful as the control he has over himself.

THE POWER OF THE BEAST

The beast is not just a symbol of a man's sexual impulse, it is part of him. It makes men capable of a larger impact. If you take care of the beast and nurture it properly, you can use its power. (Refer, again, to the Jordan Peterson quote in the last chapter.)

The "beast" represents the unstoppable human spirit, whether for good or evil. It is the incredible force that gets men to achieve the most heroic or destructive feats. The beast is beyond human force. Your impulse takes the form of a beast. Men already have the monster of their impulse inside them. Its natural tendencies are instinctive, yet we do not label them so. Most men haven't felt its sheer power yet. Stand up against it by saying no to your sexual impulse, and you will. Men just have to let it manifest itself more by not depleting it of its power.

RELATIONSHIPS

If you want to fix your relationships in life, it always starts with you. It starts with the relationship you have with the deepest parts of yourself. Meet your impulse, the beast, inside you. You may have noticed its tendencies of action, aggression, ambition, competition, production, and survival. You must work on this relationship first. You must control and own the frame in this relationship. The one thing to consider is that your beast is very strong and influential, and this means you cannot overpower it with your will. For proof, look back at the times you promised never to watch porn again—and failed.

You are like the owner of a dangerous dog. You cannot keep this beast caged up all day, so you must figure out how to live productively with it. Obviously, you don't want to let it do anything harmful or anything that you deem unacceptable to your standards. Nevertheless, you must figure out how to make this relationship work. You will have to compromise a little; however, there are benefits. It will behave on a "leash" when you have fulfilled its needs (by keeping it away from triggers and redirecting its energy). If the beast needs to run around the yard for no other reason than to burn energy, let it! But when you need it to hold back from causing harm, you are firm in your decision to keep it on a short leash. You take care of the beast. Your beast shouldn't hate you but respect you, and when you need it to unleash hell, it is at your command.

At moments we will tiptoe around to avoid waking it up. At moments we hold it back from making the impact we don't want. And in other moments, we release the beast and harness its strength. Control it, and you will have its power.

A strong man has direction in his life, and an opinion about that direction. If he isn't sure about his direction, his goal is to find one. Then he must be the leader in his life and lean into that direction in the best ways he can. This is his immediate or long-term purpose, whether that be work, projects, activities, or other goals. The man doesn't have to feel good about it, but he knows having a purpose will give him some sense of meaning and help him thrive as a man. This purpose is necessary, food for his mind and spirit. He takes the part of him that is a beast and puts it to work.

The man who redirects his power in a productive way is a man of value. His power is neither wasted nor meaningless. Even if he doesn't know his life's purpose, he knows what is an unproductive use of his energy and stays away from it. A man of high value is always ready and trained to give his greatest gift. His greatest gift is often his purpose in life or part of his purpose. For it is in giving that we are fulfilled. It is in giving our gift through the power of our impulse that we enhance our gift. This is a man's mission. To use his gift for good. This is how he expresses his gratitude to God for giving him life and making him a man: by using the power of the beast-like nature that God gave him— through giving.

Seventeen

Reclaim Your Manhood and Teach Other Men

Once you reclaim the deepest part of yourself, it is up to you to keep it alive and be a gift to the world through it. To nurture it and take care of it by taking care of yourself. Be stable emotionally because, as soon as you slip, your impulse is ready. It is always ready; therefore, you must be just as ready.

You will experience true freedom. Men are lost without a sense of themselves as men and what is natural to their core. They are lost without a world that identifies and values the unique characteristics of each gender, especially the natural impulses of men. Although you may understand what it is to embrace your manhood, your impulse holds you back from really experiencing it. Once you find and experience this freedom of your core as a man, you will be enlightened. Blind as you were when you were subject to worldly things, you can now see more clearly.

We are in the biggest pandemic for men in the world. Porn is literally in your face in social media and ads. It is more accessible than food, not to mention the sexual revolution is encouraging porn and promiscuity. Yes, I called it a pandemic. It has infected men's minds

NOBODY WANTS TO TALK ABOUT THE SECRET DESTROYER OF MEN. FATHERS DON'T TELL THEIR SONS, AND MEN DON'T TELL EACH OTHER.

and hearts, and it has taken men's lives as slaves. They are unable to be fully alive. Most importantly, it has made them weak and powerless. For those who are even a little aware, they recognize that they are not able to recover and have no idea how. It is only then they realize that this is a big problem.

It is not only a gift to be free from your impulse but to *know* there is freedom, and to be aware of it. Nobody talks about this pandemic. Nobody wants to talk about the secret destroyer of men. Fathers don't tell their sons, and men don't tell each other. Most men are not aware of the disease or the extent of the damage it has done. It takes men and makes them powerless, and it has been treated like a secret. But, in truth, it is a secret only to the people who keep it that way. This disease is worldwide, and its infectious agents are everywhere. It is advertised and extremely well publicized. I provide a plan to take back your manhood, and true self, in this book. The only other way to defeat it is to leave technology entirely—and this is not very realistic in today's technologically based world.

Once you experience this freedom, live it. Live your new life without apology. Whoever helped influence you toward freedom can never be thanked enough. You cannot repay what they have given you. That is why you pass it on. Just like parents, who give their children life. How are they supposed to repay *their* parents? That is why they pass life on to their own children.

For somebody to empower you is a true gift. For somebody to open your eyes and point you in the direction of self-empowerment through freedom is a priceless gift. This freedom doesn't empower anybody but you. Again, you cannot thank God or the people who helped you enough. They have helped give you awareness of, and freedom from, your impulse. How great is it to be able to give that gift to someone else? To empower men who need it and to give it freely without expectation.

You cannot blame men for being slaves to their impulse in today's world. How could you? The exposure and ignorance only make it expected. The boy masturbating to magazines never thought he would be begging for sexual freedom in the future because it progressively took control of his life. Most boys today are unaware of this pandemic. Their fathers don't teach them about it. Their brothers and friends don't warn them of the destructive monster it can become.

Men are not aware of the depressed and even suicidal person they can become because of their impulse. Sex and shame have become forbidden to talk about: culture has made it that way. The lack of awareness and lack of acceptance of masculinity in culture has subconsciously conditioned men to believe it to be forbidden. It may be joked about but never further discussed. Vulnerability is hard enough, plus the smart assumption that others will most likely not accept your vulnerability makes it extra hard. Most men end up believing they have to go at their impulse alone, which, as we know, can make it worse. Also, society seems to encourage your impulse. Nobody talks about these things directly, but they are implied.

Sex education implies that you cannot control your impulse, so use contraception. Nudity and vanity in magazines and online imply the encouragement of sex, and the fact that nobody talks about it implies that it is a secret and not to be discussed. Boys are growing up in a society where the only way to avoid feeding their impulse is to never leave their homes, never watch the news or TV, never play any video games, and never surf the web. Basically, don't use the Internet or technology. Since this is mostly unavoidable, boys are exposed to "suggestions" for sex . . . *all the time*. Suggestions are everywhere and so easy to access. It is not a matter of if your son or friend is exposed to porn, but when he is. Men throughout history, up to this point in time, have not had the same access to sexual stimuli in their life as we do. For men to avoid sexual stimuli, they would need to go somewhere where they would be excluded from society. They would have to get rid of their phone, their computer, their TV, and more. But even if you can block sexual content from your phone, you can also unblock it. Also, who says your impulse isn't powerful enough to get you to drive miles to access it? In today's world, access to sexual stimuli is everywhere. All you need is a phone and Internet connection.

Do not blame men for being slaves to their impulse; instead, help them. It is destroying them. It is keeping them from being much more. They did not ask for such times of slavery, but they are the case, and men can either let these times consume and destroy them or transform them. Responsibility isn't chosen; it's taken. With impulses so dark and secretive in society, it can make freedom so much sweeter.

Be the hope for your fellow victims. Men who have seen and are aware of the treacherous past of their impulse walk around and acknowledge each other like they have PTSD. Like they were fighting on the same battlefield side by side. Rapport has already been built through pain and now has the capability of creating an unstoppable brotherhood. These men that are on that battlefield today are your fathers, grandfathers, brothers, friends, and even your sons. Even the young boys enter the battlefield, unaware of what they are up against. If only they knew. If only they could go to someone. That boy was once you. Not scared when you should have been, but lacking any real place to turn.

Your recovery journey is never over, and you are never done redirecting your power as a gift. When you start to succeed in recovering, you become a leader. Not because you have the attributes of a leader, but because you are an example of what sexually impulsive slaves truly want. Freedom! Let your conviction pour outward. You can help free

> THEY DID NOT ASK FOR SUCH TIMES OF SLAVERY, BUT THEY ARE THE CASE, AND MEN CAN EITHER LET THESE TIMES CONSUME AND DESTROY THEM OR TRANSFORM THEM.

other men from their prison. You can help them take off the blind-fold so they can see the truth about their impulse. There is nothing as impactful as helping others with their impulses to solidify your own decision to recover and continue to recover.

Most men don't have a parent telling them, and helping them, to take control. And if they do, they probably don't understand the impulse as we do. So talk to your sons, your brothers, your friends, and your fathers. Expect the impulse to overcome them, but encourage them to overcome it. You can be the one other men turn to because we accept humble strength through our own understanding. You can be the one who brings up the subject because it is necessary in a society for strong men to flourish. Let us hear each other out and give advice to each other as mentors and advisers. We all have both a common challenge and common goal. It's always up to the individual person to recover; however, encouraging him through it and living out your redirection can make all the difference.

The biggest way you can influence others is by living out your gift. By letting your power magnify into your work and life. By being the one people look to for strength. Amplify this power and embrace its gift in gratitude for the people and influences you have had along your journey. Live it out and be a strong example for others.

REDEMPTION

You may be successful in recovery; however, there is always a trail behind you of your past. Maybe a trail of resentment and anger toward those who could have helped you but did not. Nevertheless, you followed a path of impulsive slavery. You have seen both the darkness of this slavery and the magnificence of freedom. Slavery was your old identity. Look back on your past, not to despise it, but to heal from it. Look back so you can forgive, learn from the experience, and move on.

Find redemption through the way you live. Redemption is found not in correcting your superiors but in being, now for others, who your superiors needed to have been for you. Men who can lead other men to freedom. Men who understand the power of their impulse and know the damage it can do. Be the kind of person you needed when you were enslaved by your impulse. Don't be afraid to bring awareness to this pandemic. To break down the social barriers keeping men from discussing their "secret." We need to make this knowledge known to every man. The longer the secret is withheld from boys and men, the more damage it does.

> *"The truth is like a lion; you don't have to defend it.*
> *Let it loose; it will defend itself."*
> —Augustine of Hippo

Men walk around today blind and not knowing what they are truly capable of. Men today are like zombies, sluggish and not as motivated and excited about things as they could be. They keep scratching the wound and making it worse. They keep falling back into the black hole of despair. It is seen as a curse on all men today; however, I see this as an opportunity for the strongest men who have ever lived.

I see a new world where the friction of transformation will create heat which will forge new bonds between men. Men all around the world will come together because they have a deeper understanding of their impulse and their power. These men may not know it, but they understand each other and the pain and struggle we all go through. For the men who have opened their eyes to see, for the men who have fought the good fight, for the men who have struggled and persevered, there are men just like you who can relate to you, who need your courage, and

MEN TODAY ARE LIKE ZOMBIES, SLUGGISH AND NOT AS MOTIVATED AND EXCITED ABOUT THINGS AS THEY COULD BE.

will also encourage you. I see a new age of strong men who open their eyes to the truth and come together to create a new world. Who redirect their power toward good and change the course of history. Not all men will be free, but the ones who fight for freedom and use it will see and experience the true capacity of their power. The power that is biologically deep in their core. The power of men.

I AM TALKING ABOUT TRUE EMPOWERMENT. A POWER THAT CANNOT BE SWAYED OR BOUGHT. A POWER WITHIN THAT MAKES YOU STRONG AND RESILIENT.

Most of us live in a world run by others. By those who seek to only empower themselves and disempower you. To them, your empowerment is a threat. I am talking about true empowerment. A power that cannot be swayed or bought. A power within that makes you strong and resilient. An energy that flows on your command that cannot be wielded by another. This power is within the biology of all men. The secret that will control men or empower them.

And yet this secret is no longer a secret. This type of impulse is no longer a detriment to your life. This impulse enhances your life; it is the inspiration deep inside you.

This is your new Super Power.

Note to Reader

Pass this book on to one man in your life, and tell him how it has impacted you.

People only retain, at most, 10 percent of what they read. I recommend reading this book at least three times. Once you more fully understand what it takes and how to overcome your impulse, it will start to become second nature to implement it.

The Hopeless Addict . . .

My addiction started and became my hope mechanism. It robs me of confidence and freedom. It deceives me of fulfillment. I want to stop, but I can't. I am powerless over it. I am tired of this disease and tired of being tired. All seems hopeless. But life moves on. I decide to pay my dues to my addiction so it doesn't freak out. It demands more and more of me. I'm afraid it will demand too much of me. It is as though I sold my soul to it and cannot take it back. I try to ignore the pain I feel from it, and that seems to get me by. I try to numb myself with it so I don't have to face the reality of my situation. I forget what freedom feels like. I am too afraid to face my addiction again. I am too afraid to be humiliated by it.

. . . A Dream

My dream is to see a world where every porn industry closes down because the operators no longer have any viewers.

Where women and men never post inappropriate pictures on social media because they know they will lose a majority of their followers.

Where sex doesn't sell—but rather deters.

Letter to Porn

DEAR PORN,

I forgive you for all the shame and hopelessness you put me through. For the insecurities you made me feel. The mental trauma of keeping you a secret because I did not know what to do or where to turn. I forgive you for the massive amounts of time and sexual power you took from me. Time that can never be taken back. Time that could have been spent giving to those I love and fueling the dreams I have for this life. I especially forgive you for the distorted view you put in my brain of what sex was and the negative effect you have had on my brain. I forgive you for manipulating me, hurting me, and enslaving me through your easy access and accessibility.

You may never understand the damage you've done. However, I am determined to end this relationship that I have relied on so much. You're right, though, about this: it was my fault for letting you. I will not be shameful of myself but will use the trauma of my experiences to better my life and that of those around me. I will redirect this power into a gift to others in the world. I will truly love the world—the trauma you have forced on me will be my fuel.

You are my dragon, and I will fiercely fight against you, for I will never again settle for slavery.

Bibliography (By Chapter)

GLOSSARY, OR DEFINITIONS OF TERMS; SOURCES INCLUDE:

Emily Ridout and Aly Rusciano, "Masculine & Feminine Energies: What They Are & How to Balance Them," last updated: May 30, 2023, https://www.wikihow.com/Masculine-vs-Feminine-Energy (accessed March 21, 2024).

Kenneth Sorensen, "Subpersonalities, According to Roberto Assagioli," 2022, https://kennethsorensen.dk/en/subpersonalities-according-to-roberto-assagioli/ (accessed March 9, 2024).

"Shit test," Urban Dictionary, August 7, 2019, https://www.urbandictionary.com/define.php?term=shit%20test (accessed Dec. 12, 2023).

Beauty For Ashes, "What Is Inner Strength? Proven Strategies to Find Your Internal Strength," December 21, 2021, https://www.bfaadvocacy.com/what-is-inner-strength/#:~:text=Inner%20strength%20simply%20means%20your%20inner%20fortitude.%20It,within%20yourself%3B%20it%20doesn%E2%80%99t%20depend%20on%20anyone%20else) (accessed Dec. 22, 2023).

Andrew Ferebee, "High-Value Man: Definition, Traits, and How to Become One", March 20, 2023, https://www.knowledgeformen.com/high-value-man/#:~:text=A%20high-value%20man%20is%20the%20

epitome%20of%20masculinity%2C,significant%20progress%20in%20
every%20part%20of%20his%20life (accessed Dec. 23, 2023).

CHAPTER 1

Napoleon Hill, *Think and Grow Rich* (New York: Ballantine Books,
1960), p. 155, 157, 171.

Rollo Tomassi, "The Rational Male Quotes," https://www.goodreads.
com/work/quotes/26430071-the-rational-male (accessed Dec. 22, 2023).

Brett McKay, "Testosterone Week: A Short Primer on How T Is Made,"
January 15, 2013, https://www.artofmanliness.com/health-fitness/
health/how-testosterone-is-made/ (accessed Dec. 12, 2023).

Joe Herbert, *Testosterone* (New York: Oxford University Press, 2015), p.
73.

Stefan Aarnio, *Hard Times Create Strong Men* (Franklin, Tenn.:
Clovercroft Publishing, 2018), p. 276, 278.

Jack Donovan, *The Way of Men* (Milwaukie, Ore.: Dissonant Hum,
2012), p. 164.

CHAPTER 2

https://www.merriam-webster.com/dictionary/power (accessed Dec. 12,
2023).

https://search.yahoo.com/search?fr=mcafee&type=E210US-
739G0&p=hypergamy&vm=r (accessed Dec. 12, 2023).

https://search.yahoo.com/search?p=highly+sexed+definition&-
fr=mcafee-s&fr2=p%3Afp%2Cm%3Asa%2Cct%3Ahistory%2Ck-
t%3Anone&ei=UTF-8&fp=1&mkr=13&vm=r (accessed Dec. 12, 2023).

CHAPTER 3

David Ludden, Ph.D., "How Men Really Feel About Pornography"
August 8, 2018, https://www.psychologytoday.com/au/blog/talking-

apes/201808/how-men-really-feel-about-pornography (accessed Dec. 12, 2023).

Melinda Wenner, "Why Do Guys Get Sleepy After Sex?" February 1, 2013. https://www.livescience.com/32445-why-do-guys-get-sleepy-after-sex.html (accessed Dec. 12, 2023).

Max Jones, "Pornographic Weaponization Against the Palestinians By Israel," March 11, 2023. https://medium.com/@tsyaochyaoi/pornographic-weaponization-against-the-palestinians-by-israel-4b5f29992f28 (accessed March 18, 2024).

Herbert A. Friedman, "Looking Back: Sex in Psychological Warfare", January 20, 2009. https://www.bps.org.uk/psychologist/looking-back-sex-psychological-warfare (accessed March 18, 2024).

Daniel Haqiqatjou, "Pornography as Israel's Weapon of Choice," January 10, 2019. https://muslimskeptic.com/2019/01/10/pornography-israel-weapon-of-war/ (accessed March 18, 2024).

Four chemicals are referenced in this chapter: oxytocin, prolactin, vasopressin, serotonin:

Cleveland Clinic, "Oxytocin: What It Is, Function & Effects." Last reviewed by a Cleveland Clinic medical professional on 03/27/2022. https://my.clevelandclinic.org/health/articles/22618-oxytocin#additional-common-questions (accessed Dec. 12, 2023).

BetterHelp, "What Are The Effects Of Oxytocin On Men?" October 16, 2023, medically reviewed by Julie Dodson. https://www.betterhelp.com/advice/medication/what-is-the-role-of-oxytocin-in-men/ (accessed Dec. 12, 2023).

Ruo-Bing Teng, Xin-Hua Zhang, "Oxytocin and male sexual function," June 17, 2011, https://pubmed.ncbi.nlm.nih.gov/21735659/ (accessed Dec. 12, 2023).

Tomas, "Symptoms and Treatment for High Prolactin in Men" November 21, 2021, https://www.ourhairstyle.com/symptoms-and-treatment-for-high-prolactin-in-men/ (accessed Dec. 12, 2023).

Andrea Cooper, "What Is a Prolactin Test?" Medically reviewed by Jabeen Begum, MD, on Dec. 14, 2023. https://www.webmd.com/a-to-z-guides/prolactin-test (accessed Dec. 22, 2023).

Cleveland Clinic, "Prolactin", by a Cleveland Clinic medical professional on February 15, 2022. https://my.clevelandclinic.org/health/articles/22429-prolactin#resources (accessed Dec. 12, 2023).

Times Mojo, "Does Prolactin Decrease Dopamine?", July 7, 2022. https://www.timesmojo.com/does-prolactin-decrease-dopamine/#:~:text=Prolactin%20plays%20an%20important%20role%20in%20maternal%20behavior.,sex%20hormones%E2%80%94estrogen%20in%20women%20and%20testosterone%20in%20men (accessed Dec. 12, 2023).

David Jaynes, "High Prolactin Low Testosterone", https://morningsteel.com/high-prolactin-low-testosterone/ (accessed Dec. 12, 2023).

Cathy Cassata, "What Is Vasopressin?", Medically reviewed by Kacy Church, MD, September 22, 2023. https://www.everydayhealth.com/vasopressin/guide/ (accessed Dec. 12, 2023).

M. Nadal, "Secretory rhythm of vasopressin in healthy subjects with inversed sleep—wake cycle: evidence for the existence of an intrinsic regulation", February 1996, https://pubmed.ncbi.nlm.nih.gov/8630515/#:~:text=It%20was%20concluded%20that%20the%20secretion%20of%20vasopressin,nor%20to%20variations%20in%20plasma%20osmolality%20or%20electrolytes (accessed Dec. 12, 2023).

Angelica Bottaro, "What Is Serotonin?" Updated on October 26, 2023. https://www.verywellhealth.com/what-is-serotonin-5189485 (accessed Dec. 12, 2023).

Stefan Aarnio, *Hard Times Create Strong Men* (Franklin, Tenn.: Clovercroft Publishing, 2018), p. 275.

CHAPTER 4

Stefan Aarnio, *Hard Times Create Strong Men* (Franklin, Tenn.: Clovercroft Publishing, 2018), p. 275.

Shivali Best, "Children who watch pornography at a young age are more likely to have sex earlier and adopt 'unhealthy sexual habits' later in life" Sept. 6, 2017.

https://www.dailymail.co.uk/sciencetech/article-4858590/Kids-watch-porn-young-age-likely-sex.html (accessed Dec. 12, 2023).

Karla Hamlen, "Re-examining Gender Differences in Video Game Play: Time Spent and Feelings of Success." October 2010. https://www.researchgate.net/publication/254582197_Re-Examining_Gender_Differences_in_Video_Game_Play_Time_Spent_and_Feelings_of_Success#:~:text=The%20current%20study%20shows%20that%2C%20when%20accounting%20for,and%20achievement%2C%20which%20then%20prompts%20more%20time%20playing (accessed Dec. 12, 2023).

Forbes, "The World's Highest-Paid Athletes." 2022: https://www.forbes.com/athletes/list/#tab:overall (accessed Dec. 12, 2022).

Mark Cartwright, "Roman Gladiator." May 3, 2018. https://www.world-history.org/gladiator/ (accessed Dec. 12, 2023).

Christian-Georges Schwentzel, "Did the Romans and Greeks really enjoy orgies?" August 2, 2023. https://theconversation.com/did-the-romans-and-greeks-really-enjoy-orgies-210736 (accessed Dec. 12, 2023).

Evan Andrews, "8 Reasons Why Rome Fell," January 14, 2014. https://www.history.com/news/8-reasons-why-rome-fell (accessed Jan. 23, 2024).

Nancy Schimelpfening, "Emotional Blunting: Causes, Symptoms & Treatment." Updated on November 6, 2023. https://www.verywellmind.com/can-antidepressants-make-you-feel-emotionally-numb-1067348 (accessed Jan. 23, 2024).

Yahoo, "masculinity" https://search.yahoo.com/search?-fr2=p%3ads%2cv%3aomn%2cm%3asa%2cbrws%3achrome%2cpos-%3a2&fr=mcafee&type=E210US739G0&p=masculinity+defini-tion&vm=r (accessed Dec. 12, 2023).

Phillip Noyce, "The Giver", 2014. https://www.imdb.com/title/tt0435651/ (accessed Dec. 12, 2023).

Shale Marks, LCSW CADC and Dr. Kimberly Dennis, MD, "Baby Elephant Beliefs," August 12, 2018.

https://suncloudhealth.com/blog/baby-elephant-beliefs-written-shale-marks-lcsw-cadc-dr-kimberly-dennis-md#:~:text=There%E2%80%99s%20an%20old%20adage%20about%20baby%20elephants.%20Circus,in%20the%20ground%2C%20still%20believed%20it%20couldn%E2%80%99t%20move (accessed Jan. 23, 2024).

FirstVet, "What You Need to Know About Neutering Your Male Dog." September 2020. https://firstvet.com/us/articles/what-you-need-to-know-about-neutering-your-male-dog#:~:text=The%20best-known%20benefit%20of%20neutering%20a%20male%20dog,age%20often%20have%20fewer%20problems%20with%20testosterone-related%20behaviors (accessed Dec. 12, 2023).

Krysten Crawford, "New Stanford education study shows where boys and girls do better in math, English," June 13, 2018. https://ed.stanford.edu/news/new-stanford-education-study-shows-where-boys-and-girls-do-better-math-english#:~:text=Girls%20surpass%20boys%20on%20reading%20and%20writing%20in,grade%2C%20girls%20are%20almost%20a%20full%20grade%20ahead (accessed Dec. 12, 2023).

Heather Jones, "Do ADHD Symptoms Differ in Boys and Girls?" Updated on June 1, 2023. https://www.verywellhealth.com/do-adhd-symptoms-differ-in-boys-and-girls-5207995 (accessed Dec. 12, 2023).

Marjo, "It's Illegal for Students to Play This Gym Class Game in Massachusetts Schools." Updated on June 1, 2023. https://www.verywellhealth.com/do-adhd-symptoms-differ-in-boys-and-girls-5207995 (accessed Dec. 12, 2023).

Joe Herbert, *Testosterone* (New York: Oxford University Press, 2015), p. 82.

Jonah Berger, "Social Conformity—Brain Games," Dec. 14, 2015. https://www.youtube.com/watch?v=o8BkzvP19v4 (accessed Dec. 12, 2023).

CHAPTER 5

Stefan Aarnio, *Hard Times Create Strong Men* (Franklin, Tenn.: Clovercroft Publishing, 2018).

CHAPTER 6

David Fincher, *Fight Club*, 1999. David Flincher, director; writers: Chuck Palahniuk, Jim Uhls. https://www.imdb.com/title/tt0137523/?ref_%3Dref_ext_justwatch (accessed Dec. 12, 2023).

Stephanie Osmanski, "Enjoy the 70 Best 'Fight Club' Quotes, and Let the Chips Fall Where They May"; Updated: Sept. 20, 2023. https://parade.com/movies/fight-club-quotes (accessed Dec. 12, 2023).

Chuck Palahniuk, "Chuck Palahniuk, Fight Club." https://www.goodreads.com/quotes/136976-remember-this-the-people-you-re-trying-to-step-on-we-re (accessed Dec. 12, 2023).

CHAPTER 7

Abbey Rennemeyer, "The 80-20 Rule: The Pareto Principle Explained in Plain English," December 28, 2020. https://www.freecodecamp.org/news/the-80-20-rule-pareto-principle-explained-in-plain-english/ (accessed Dec. 12, 2023).

Sabrina Talbert, "Does Birth Control Stop Your Period? Experts Share Everything You Need To Know," Nov. 29, 2022. https://www.womenshealthmag.com/health/a41981749/does-birth-control-stop-your-period/ (accessed Dec. 12, 2023).

Andi Breitowich, "Why Is My Period So Light? 9 Potential Reasons, According To Ob-Gyns," Jan. 23, 2024. https://www.womenshealthmag.com/health/a46353560/why-is-my-period-so-light/ (accessed Jan. 28, 2024).

Napoleon Hill, *Think and Grow Rich* (New York: Ballantine Books, 1960), p. 175.

CHAPTER 8

David Deida, *The Way of the Superior Man.* (Boulder, Colo.: Sounds True, Inc., 1997), pp. 3-4.

Sexaholics Anonymous literature, Sexaholics Anonymous (1989), p. 24.

Amanda Onion, Missy Sullivan, Matt Mullen, and Christian Zapata. "Plato", November 9, 2009. https://www.history.com/topics/ancient-greece/plato (accessed Jan. 28, 2024).

Corey Wayne, "Attraction Is Not a Choice," April 19, 2015. https://understandingrelationships.com/attraction-is-not-a-choice/19521 (accessed Jan. 28, 2024).

Corey Wayne, "She's Totally Above Me. She's Out of My League," November 18, 2021. https://coachcoreywayne.medium.com/shes-totally-above-me-she-s-out-of-my-league-f2eb92e2badf (accessed Jan. 28, 2024).

Dr. NerdLove, "Do You Suffer from Oneitis?", September 9, 2011. https://www.doctornerdlove.com/oneitis/(accessed Jan. 28, 2024).

Corey Wayne, "The Importance of Sharing the Same Values," April 27, 2022. https://coachcoreywayne.medium.com/the-importance-of-sharing-the-same-values-97dd1c591e3. (accessed Jan. 28, 2024).

Rollo Tomassi, *The Rational Male.* https://www.goodreads.com/quotes/10052052-in-any-relationship-the-person-with-the-most-power-is (accessed Dec. 12, 2023).

New American Bible, Revised Edition

Timothy A Carey Ph.D. "Actions Don't Speak Louder Than Words." August 1, 2022. https://www.psychologytoday.com/us/blog/in-control/202208/actions-dont-speak-louder-words (accessed Dec. 12, 2023).

Muise, Amy, Schimmack, Ulrich, Impett, Emily. "Sexual Frequency Predicts Greater Well-Being, But More Is Not Always Better" (2015).

Social Psychological and Personality Science. https://www.researchgate.
net/publication/284175688_Sexual_Frequency_Predicts_Greater_Well-
Being_But_More_is_Not_Always_Better (accessed Dec. 12, 2023).

Carol Church, "Will Having More Sex Improve Your Relationship?"
June 22, 2020. https://smartcouples.ifas.ufl.edu/married/sex-and-inti-
macy/will-having-more-sex-improve-your-relationship/ (accessed Jan.
28, 2024).

Collins Dictionary, "flirtation," https://www.collinsdictionary.com/dic-
tionary/english/flirtation (accessed Jan. 28, 2024).

Charlotte Howard, "Compromise Vs. Negotiation in Couples
Counseling," Austin, Texas https://deepeddypsychotherapy.com/
compromise-negotiation-couples-counseling/ (accessed Jan.
28, 2024). Also as a YouTube video at: https://m.youtube.com/
watch?time_continue=133&v=_vBy6sE5gBU&embeds_refer-
ring_euri=https%3A%2F%2Fdeepeddypsychotherapy.com%2Fcom-
promise-negotiation-couples-counseling%2F&source_ve_path=N-
zY3NTg&feature=emb_yt_watermark (accessed Jan. 28, 2024).

Cleveland Clinic, "Blue Balls: Facts and Fiction," January 17,
2023. https://health.clevelandclinic.org/blue-balls (accessed Jan. 28,
2024).

Viney Dhiman, "10 Benefits of Semen Retention That Turn You Into
Alpha Male," November 30, 2021. https://ladtribe.com/semen-reten-
tion-benefits/ (accessed Jan. 28, 2024).

Deb Levine, MA, Stephanie Watson, "Sex Pheromones: What Are These
Chemical Messengers?" November 3, 2023. https://www.webmd.com/
sex-relationships/sex-life-pheromones (accessed Jan. 28, 2024).

Rahul Gambhir, "Semen Retention: Is It Harmful? Plus Benefits, Side
Effects & More," February 23, 2021. https://manmatters.com/blog/what-
is-semen-retention-benefits-side-effects-more/ (accessed Jan. 28, 2024).

CHAPTER 9

C.S. Lewis, "Quote By C.S. Lewis," https://www.goodreads.com/quotes/116204-only-know-how-strong (accessed Jan. 28, 2024).

Joe Herbert, *Testosterone* (New York: Oxford University Press, 2015), p. 37.

Sexaholics Anonymous literature, Sexaholics Anonymous (1989), pp. 4; 87.

Genesis 50:20, https://www.bible.com/bible/3034/GEN.50.20.BSB (accessed Jan. 28, 2024).

Confucius, "Quotes By Confucius," https://www.goodreads.com/quotes/465597-the-man-who-says-he-can-and-the-man-who (accessed Jan. 28, 2024).

Napoleon Hill, *Think and Grow Rich* (New York: Ballantine Books, 1960), p. 17.

Brett and Kate McKay, "8 Interesting (And Insane) Male Rites of Passages from Around the World," February 21, 2010. https://www.artofmanliness.com/character/behavior/male-rites-of-passage-from-around-the-world/ (accessed Feb. 2, 2024).

Christopher Nolan, director, *Batman Begins,* 2005, https://www.imdb.com/title/tt0372784/ (accessed Dec. 12, 2023).

J.D. Meier, "How Tony Robbins Transformed His Life with Goals," Copyright © 2024. https://sourcesofinsight.com/how-tony-robbins-transformed-his-life-with-goals/ (accessed Feb. 2, 2024).

CHAPTER 10

Tony Robbins, "Tony Robbins Quotes About Pain," 2012, https://www.azquotes.com/author/12429-Tony_Robbins/tag/pain (accessed Feb. 2, 2024).

CHAPTER 11

Napoleon Hill, "Napoleon Hill Quotes," https://www.goodreads.com/author/quotes/399.Napoleon_Hill?page=27 (accessed Dec. 12, 2023).

The Holy Bible, New International Version, Matthew 16:25. https://biblehub.com/matthew/16-25.htm (accessed Dec. 12, 2023).

CHAPTER 12

Fr. Mike Schmitz, "What Does Surrender Actually Look Like?" May 19, 2021. https://www.youtube.com/watch?v=aabwei87sQM (accessed Dec. 12, 2023).

Kelly McClanahan, "What Does 'Surrender' Really Mean?" November 21, 2014. https://www.soberrecovery.com/recovery/surrender/ (accessed Feb. 2, 2024).

CHAPTER 13

David Deida, *The Way of the Superior Man* (Boulder, Colo.: Sounds True, Inc., 1997), p. 48.

CHAPTER 14

Sexaholics Anonymous literature, Sexaholics Anonymous (1989), p. 24.

Dr. NerdLove, "Do You Suffer from Oneitis?", September 9, 2011. https://www.doctornerdlove.com/oneitis/(accessed Jan. 28, 2024).

Christopher M. Osborne, PhD, "How to End an Erection," May 17, 2023. https://www.wikihow.com/End-an-Erection (accessed Feb. 9, 2024).

CHAPTER 15

Cornell University, Richard P. Riney, "What Are Zoomies?" 2016. https://www.vet.cornell.edu/departments/riney-canine-health-center/canine-health-information/what-are-zoomies (accessed Dec. 12, 2023)

David Deida, *The Way of the Superior Man* (Boulder, Colo.: Sounds True, Inc., 1997), pp. 131, 148.

The Holy Bible, New International Version, Revelation 3:16. https://bible-hub.com/revelation/3-16.htm (accessed Feb. 9, 2024).

Jordan Peterson, "Jordan Peterson Quotes," Jan 30, 2018. https://jordan-petersonquotes.com/you-should-be-a-monster/ (accessed Feb. 9, 2024).

Andrew Ferebee, "9 Masculinity Traits That Change Boys into Men," June 7, 2023. https://www.knowledgeformen.com/masculini-ty-traits/ (accessed Feb. 9, 2024).

CHAPTER 16

Exton MS, Krüger TH, Bursch N, Haake P, Knapp W, Schedlowski M, Hartmann U. "Endocrine response to masturbation-induced orgasm in healthy men following a 3-week sexual abstinence." November 19, 2001. https://pubmed.ncbi.nlm.nih.gov/11760788/ (accessed Dec. 12, 2023).

Rahul Gambhir, "Semen Retention: Is It Harmful? Plus Benefits, Side Effects & More," February 23, 2021. https://manmatters.com/blog/what-is-semen-retention-benefits-side-effects-more/ (accessed Dec. 12, 2023).

Diane McGee, "17 Benefits of Semen Retention You Probably Don't Know About," November 28, 2022. https://www.formatex.info/bene-fits-of-semen-retention/ (accessed Feb. 9, 2024).

Anubhav Bhatt, "22+ Semen Retention Benefits to PROVE Why You Need It!", September 21, 2023. https://menverve.com/22-semen-reten-tion-benefits/#deeper-emotional-connection (accessed Feb. 9, 2024).

CHAPTER 17

Augustine of Hippo, "Quote by Augustine of Hippo." https://www.goodreads.com/quotes/798196-the-truth-is-like-a-lion-you-don-t-have-to (accessed Dec. 12, 2023).